ADDICTION
IS
ADDICTION

WORKBOOK

Understanding the disease in oneself
and others for a better quality of life

— by —
Sue Newton
Paige Abbott
Raju Hajela

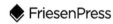 FriesenPress

Suite 300 - 990 Fort St
Victoria, BC, V8V 3K2
Canada

www.friesenpress.com

ISBN
978-1-5255-1509-5 (Hardcover)
978-1-5255-1510-1 (Paperback)
978-1-5255-1511-8 (eBook)

1. SELF-HELP, SUBSTANCE ABUSE & ADDICTIONS

Distributed to the trade by The Ingram Book Company

Table of Contents

Acknowledgements

We would like to express our gratitude to all those who have read our book *Addiction is Addiction* and encouraged us to write this practical workbook.

We would like to thank our patients, family and friends for their encouragement and feedback about our work that continues to enhance the understanding of Addiction and mental health-related problems, in the context of improving our individual lives together with supporting healthier families and communities.

A special thank you to Martin C. and Paul St. R. for reading the initial draft of our workbook and providing us with their valuable feedback. We would also like to thank Dr. Stephen Karpman for granting us permission to use the Karpman Drama Triangle in our text, which we have adapted to explain some important issues related to the dysfunctional traps that can be present in relationships and develop constructs related to dealing with the dysfunctions.

We would like to acknowledge the Foundation for Addiction and Mental Health (FAMH) (www.famh.ca). FAMH is a grassroots community-based charitable organization committed to sharing the reality about Addiction and mental health, the potential links between Addiction and other secondary health conditions, and the continuing care required for long term recovery. As with our book *Addiction is Addiction,* we will continue to donate some of the workbook sale proceeds to support FAMH.

Introduction

Our goal in writing this workbook is to help you appreciate the principles discussed in our book, *Addiction is Addiction*, and to expand your awareness and provide clarity about how the disease has been affecting you and others around you. It is helpful, although not necessary to have read *Addiction is Addiction* prior to starting this workbook. This resource has been designed for those who have read our previous book and those who have not.

For those who have read our book, you will find some intentional repetition of concepts to provide consistency and background for the questions and activities proposed in this workbook. For new readers, we have attempted to capture enough background information to complete the activities but if you feel you need more information, we recommend reading our book.

In each chapter there will be a combination of information to enhance knowledge as well as relevant questions and activities to generate introspection and take action. Throughout the workbook, a break will be recommended in an effort to allow you to rest and assimilate the information and activities in the previous sections. The recommended breaks will be identified by the HUM logo:

We also hope that this workbook will help you apply these principles in your daily life to ensure that recovery becomes the top priority. Even though you may have picked up this workbook to see how you could help someone else with substance-related or addiction-related problems, it would be very important to go through this workbook for yourself.

In Chapter 1, we will explore your current views and understanding of Addiction as well as common beliefs. The difference between substance abuse versus Addiction will be discussed and Addiction beyond substances will be introduced. We will introduce the concept of genetic predisposition and at the end of this chapter, the activity will be to draw your family tree to identify who you think may have or had addiction-related problems. Mapping your ancestry on a family tree is a great way to help understand your heritage and genetic history as well as gain knowledge about extended family members you may or may not have met.

In Chapter 2, we will explain what makes Addiction a primary, chronic brain disease—meaning it is not caused by something else and it is lifelong. Once someone has Addiction, it does not go away and people need recovery to deal with the disease to optimize their health and well-being. Addiction is influenced by both genetics and environment, similar to other chronic diseases such as Diabetes and Cardiovascular Disease. Simply put, a disease is a malfunction of one or more organs in the body and brain and is typically manifested by distinguishing symptoms and characteristics that are common in all the people who have that disease. With Addiction, that organ that is malfunctioning is the brain. All of us are hardwired with a reward circuitry in our midbrain that is designed to make food (eating) and sex desirable activities in our lives. We need food to survive and sex to procreate, and so the human brain is designed to make these pleasurable. Anytime something feels good, there is a release of the neurotransmitter dopamine, together with other chemicals, to reinforce that behaviour, to increase the likelihood in repeating or seeking that activity again. So each of us is vulnerable to seeking what feels good, which with Addiction can take a life of its own, with no off switch, because of our genetics, brain function, environment, and exposure to substances and unhealthy behaviours. The questions and exercises in this chapter will help you better understand the disease.

Increasing awareness and understanding of addictive thinking, feeling, and behaviour is critical for everyone impacted by Addiction because they are indicators of how active the disease is and if a person is engaging in healthy recovery. As Addiction is a chronic disease that lasts a lifetime, there can be periods of relapse and remission. Being in tune with addictive thinking, feeling, and behaviours is important in mitigating relapse. There is more in-depth discussion on this is in Chapters 3 through 5, in which we discuss addictive thinking, feeling, and behaviours. The questions and exercises will help you appreciate these better in your life and those you love.

In Chapter 6, our focus shifts from the disease of Addiction to holistic recovery with an emphasis on a bio-psycho-social-spiritual perspective. This chapter looks at the important components of recovery including self-management, peer and professional support. We discuss setting goals, willingness, and the essentials of continuing care by looking at Addiction as a chronic, lifelong disease. The questions and exercises will help you develop a personalized recovery plan.

In Chapter 7, we introduce you to RAiAR, a relatively new platform for recovery. RAiAR stands for *Remember Addiction is Addiction Responsible Recovery*. RAiAR is a mutual support program, which offers weekly, closed, small group meetings with occasional speaker meetings, to assist people in recovery from Addiction.

In Chapter 8, we focus on family issues to help you become aware of common family roles people fall into. We will discuss the importance of assertiveness, boundaries, emotional healing, and healthy communication with sample scenarios for practice. We will also clarify independence versus interdependence, which honours each person's unique identity, while recognizing that we all need to rely on each other in a healthy way.

Chapter 9 is the summary and conclusion section. We end off with an Appendix to provide more information about RAiAR and resources for further reading and learning.

As this workbook is a practical complement to our book, *Addiction is Addiction*, the title remains the same to highlight the many facets the disease of Addiction. Throughout the workbook, we have decided to capitalize the diagnosis of Addiction rather than writing 'addiction'. This is to emphasize that Addiction, a proper noun, is the name of a serious disease. It is not to be taken lightly as Addiction can cause disability or premature death, especially when left untreated or treated inadequately.

We hope that the workbook will get you started on the exciting journey of learning about Addiction and mental health problems in yourself and those you love. The intention is to ensure a healthier relationship with your 'self' despite the nature and severity of problems you may or may not have.

Chapter 1: Understanding Addiction

"It is not our differences that divide us. It is our inability to recognize, accept, and celebrate those differences."
–Audre Lorde

What is Addiction?

As you start this workbook, we would like to begin by exploring your current beliefs and ideas about Addiction. As Addiction is a word that means different things to different people, it is essential for you to explore what it has meant to you before you can appreciate the reality of what it does mean in context of the current scientific research and best medical practice for assessment, treatment, and recovery.

What does Addiction mean to you? Is it:

Bad choices? (Place an X next to your answer)
Yes_____ No_____

Someone else's fault?
Yes_____No_____If yes, who?_____

Just excessive substance use?
Yes_____ No_____

Caused by something else? (e.g., trauma)
Yes_____No_____

Being selfish?
Yes_____ No_____

Different kinds of Addictions (e.g., food addiction, drug addiction, gambling addiction)?
Yes_____ No_____

Common beliefs about Addiction that are *not* true include:

- It is just bad behaviour or a vice
- It is self-medication
- Just wanting to get 'high'
- Making wrong or bad choices
- Just excessive substance use, "everyone does it"

- Being selfish, irresponsible
- Caused by something else (e.g., trauma)
- There are "good Addictions and bad Addictions"
- It is 'addictions' rather than 'Addiction'
- People are addicted to…..(e.g. alcohol, sex, gambling)

Addiction is a primary, chronic disease of brain reward, motivation, memory and related circuitry. This will be discussed in detail in the next chapter after you have had a chance to continue exploring your beliefs about Addiction.

"Addiction is a primary, chronic disease of brain reward, motivation, memory and related circuitry."

Are substance abuse and Addiction the same thing?

Substance abuse is an old concept that is increasingly being replaced by the term 'unhealthy substance use.' It consists of hazardous use (episodic) or harmful use (more continuous). Addiction, on the other hand, is characterized by impairment in behavioural control among other things. Although we often think of behaviour being largely driven by choice, when Addiction is involved, the choice is gone.

What substances have you used throughout your life, in any quantity? List them here.

_____

_____

_____

_____

_____

What substances have you used in your life for escape, reward, and/or relief from pain, stress, boredom, self, others, or anything else? List them here.

_____

_____

_____

_____

_____

When have you felt you had control about how much you used? Describe the feelings and situations in which this occurred.

_____

_____

_____

_____

_____

When have you not had control about how much or when you used these substances? Describe the feelings and situations in which this occurred.

_____

_____

_____

_____

_____

_____

_____

What have these substances done for you? How has this changed over time?

_____
_____
_____
_____
_____
_____

What harms may have resulted by the use of substances:
To me?

_____
_____
_____
_____
_____
_____

To others?

_____
_____
_____
_____
_____

Addiction is not just about alcohol and drugs. Many people have impaired control with food, gambling, relationships, love, fantasy, sex, video games, exercise, work, and other behaviours.

What behaviours have you used in your life for escape, reward, and/or relief from pain, stress, boredom, self, others, or anything else?

_____
_____
_____
_____
_____

When have you felt you had control about how much you used these behaviours? Describe the feelings and situations in which this occurred.

_____
_____
_____
_____
_____
_____

*When have you **not** had control about how much or when you used these behaviours? Describe the feelings and situations in which this occurred.*

_____

_____

_____

_____

_____

_____

What have these behaviours done for you? How has this changed over time?

_____

_____

_____

_____

_____

What harms may have resulted by the use of these behaviours:
To me?

_____

_____

_____

_____

_____

To others?

_____

_____

_____

_____

_____

The role of Genetics and family heritage

A genetic predisposition (also called genetic susceptibility) is an increased likelihood of developing a particular disease based on a person's genetic makeup. A genetic predisposition results from specific genetic variations that are often inherited from a parent. Some people with a predisposing genetic vulnerability may never manifest the disease while others will, even within the same family. In people with a significant genetic predisposition, the risk of disease can be aggravated by other factors, which includes lifestyle and environmental factors. Although a person's genetic makeup cannot be altered, some lifestyle and environmental modifications (e.g., abstaining from mood altering substances until age 25 or older or growing up in a household with others in healthy recovery) may be able to reduce disease risk in people with a genetic predisposition such that complications of the disease are prevented.

> *"In people with a significant genetic predisposition, the risk of disease can be aggravated by other factors, which includes lifestyle and environmental factors."*

Please draw a family tree to identify Addiction-related problems. It would be important to identify grandparents, their siblings and cousins as well as parents, their siblings and their children (your cousins and their children), in addition to your own siblings and children if applicable. Indicate on the tree using a small check mark beside the name of the individual who had or you suspect may have had Addiction-related problems. You can indicate other mental health related problems (which may be misdiagnosed or misunderstood) using an 'm' to identify those who had or you have heard had other mental health conditions or challenges.

When the genetic predisposition is strong, even the initiation of substance use is not necessarily done by choice (meaning first time using). Losing the ability to make healthy choices in Addiction means that, despite one's best intentions, the substance use and problem behaviours persist, thus aggravating the disease. Focusing solely on stopping certain behaviours or substance use can aggravate them, whereas attention to healthier behaviours in the context of the pursuit of abstinence reinforces recovery.

How do you feel about the information contained in your family tree?

_____

_____

_____

_____

_____

_____

What are some things you do to stay healthy?

_____

_____

_____

_____

_____

_____

As already mentioned, none of us can change our genetic vulnerability but we can change how we choose to live our life and choose recovery. There will be in-depth discussion on holistic recovery in Chapter 6.

The disease of "more"

The need for more and ever-increasing desires that can never be totally fulfilled are a hallmark feature of Addiction. The chase for more and the preoccupation to fulfill the persistent desires becomes the most important aspect of the person's life. All other responsibilities are neglected and daily life starts to unravel and become increasingly unmanageable. This can occur with alcohol, drugs, food, sex, relationships, gambling, fantasy, money/wealth, video games, shopping, exercise, success, and any other behaviour that becomes compulsive and unhealthy.

List examples of where you have or currently feel you need more and cannot seem to get enough:

_____

_____

_____

_____

_____

_____

For individuals who are struggling to identify whether they have Addiction or not, looking at the pursuit of 'more' and never feeling satisfied or that you have enough or are good enough are key features of Addiction. If you are experiencing these, learning more about Addiction and pursuing recovery would be essential.

Key points

- Addiction can mean different things to different people based on their past experience and beliefs

- Addiction is not synonymous to substance abuse

- Genetics plays a key role

- Addiction can manifest beyond substances with unhealthy, compulsive behaviors

- Addiction is the disease of more

Action steps for Chapter 1 (follow through after chapter exercises)

In this chapter, you began exploring your current beliefs and perceptions regarding Addiction and your own genetic predisposition. If you have not had an opportunity to talk to a family member or do not know if other family members may have Addiction-related problems, and if this is an option available to you we encourage you to ask someone in your family that may know. Family members may struggle to be honest about this and, if so, you can talk to others in your life about your feelings and intuition about your family history and health.

Chapter 2: Addiction as a Primary, Chronic Brain Disease

"When we least expect it, life sets us a challenge to test our courage and willingness to change;
at such a moment, there is no point in pretending that nothing has happened or in saying
that we are not yet ready. The challenge will not wait. Life does not look back."
—Paulo Coelho

This chapter provides more in-depth information about Addiction to increase your awareness and understanding. Without awareness, it is hard to take appropriate action. Addiction resides in the brain, so we will start off looking at how our brain impacts behaviour.

The Brain and Behaviour

All of our behaviour is the result of brain function, which affects perception, memory, motivation, learning, and action. The brain is the most complex organ in the human body and remains the most misunderstood. What we commonly call the mind is a manifestation of a set of operations carried out by the brain. Its actions underlie not only motor behaviours such as walking or talking, but also all the complex cognitive actions such as thoughts, feelings, and perceptions. Problem behaviours arise when one part of the brain is under- or over-functioning. This can produce common symptoms such as: irritability, impulsivity, compulsivity, obsession, hyperactivity, anxiety, and depression. The signs and symptoms can manifest in behavioural problems as well, which can lead to a psychiatric diagnosis and medications. The medications may mask or suppress the symptoms, but may not necessarily address the root problem in brain function that go beyond a chemical imbalance.

Addiction, by definition, is:

- *A primary, chronic disease*

- *About brain dysfunction*

- *About pathologically seeking reward*

- *About memory distortion*

- *About seeking relief*

- *About neglecting self*

- *About motivation problems*

- *About distortions in thinking, feeling, and perception*

- *About impaired behavioural control*

What do you agree with in the above? Where does that understanding come from?

_____

_____

_____

_____

_____

What do you disagree with? Where does that disagreement come from?

_____

_____

_____

_____

_____

In Addiction, behaviours are not the disease, nor do they cause it. Behaviours are a manifestation of brain function, a consequence of increased or decreased activity in specific regions of the brain. Brain function is impacted by both genetic predisposition and damage resulting from the use of alcohol, drugs, and compulsive behaviors. This perspective on brain function focuses on the biological part of the problems and hopefully will allow people to get away from the stigma and shame related to 'it is all in your head' or somehow the individual's fault in making bad choices. One must appreciate that since the brain is what one uses to make sense of whatever is happening within and around us, we would not know if or when our brain is providing misinformation due to some dysfunction.

Areas of the brain impacted by Addiction that affect behaviour include the limbic system and the pre-frontal cortex. In a healthy brain, the functions of the pre-frontal cortex are:

- *to regulate attention span*
- *perseverance*
- *judgement*
- *impulse control*
- *learning from past experiences*
- *ability to have feelings, especially empathy*

- *organization*
- *self-monitoring and supervision*
- *problem solving*
- *critical thinking*
- *forward thinking*

Problems in the pre-frontal cortex will result in:

- ☐ *short attention span*
- ☐ *distractibility*
- ☐ *lack of perseverance*
- ☐ *impulse control problems*
- ☐ *hyperactivity*
- ☐ *chronic lateness, poor time management*
- ☐ *disorganization*

- ☐ *procrastination*
- ☐ *unavailability of emotions*
- ☐ *misperceptions*
- ☐ *poor judgement*
- ☐ *trouble learning from experience*
- ☐ *short term memory problems*
- ☐ *social and test anxiety*

What symptoms have you experienced from the list above (place a check mark in the appropriate boxes)? When and how have these symptoms impacted your life?

_____

_____

_____

_____

_____

_____

_____

In a healthy brain, the functions of the limbic system are to:

- *set the emotional tone of the mind through filtering of old memories*
- *filter external events through internal states (emotional colouring)*
- *tag events as internally important or not based on past experience*

- *store highly charged emotional memories*
- *regulate motivation*
- *control appetite and sleep cycles*
- *promote bonding and attachment*
- *directly process the sense of smell*
- *regulate libido (sex drive)*

Problems in the limbic system will result in:

- ☐ *moodiness*
- ☐ *irritability*
- ☐ *clinical depression*
- ☐ *increased dysfunctional thinking*
- ☐ *perceiving events in a negative way*
- ☐ *decreased motivation*

- ☐ *flood of uncomfortable emotions*
- ☐ *change in appetite*
- ☐ *sleep problems*
- ☐ *decreased or increased sexual responsiveness*
- ☐ *social isolation*

What symptoms have you experienced from the list above (place a check mark in the appropriate boxes)? When and how have these symptoms impacted your life?

_____
_____
_____
_____
_____
_____
_____

"These symptoms are an indicator that your brain is in an unhealthy state ."

If and when you experience any of the symptoms listed above such as hyperactivity, irritability, and decreased motivation, it is important to reflect on what is currently going on in your life. These symptoms are an indicator that your brain is in an unhealthy state, which is helpful information as you pursue recovery and you start to appreciate your vulnerabilities. Are you still using any mood altering substances? Engaging in compulsive, unhealthy behaviors? Have you been triggered by your environment, exposure or stress?

The limbic system and the pre-frontal cortex are connected to the hypothalamus, the key location of the reward circuitry. If there are problems with the reward circuitry, reward and/or relief seeking is triggered through the use of substances and other behaviours, which becomes more dysfunctional when driven by alcohol and other drugs, or addictive behaviours such as eating disorders, sexual acting out, gambling or many others.

The common feature in all aspects of Addiction is the desire to escape reality through wanting more of even necessary behaviours, such as sleep, food, shopping, exercise, or work, as reality feels overwhelming or does not match the fantasy that is generated by dysfunction in brain circuits related to reward, motivation, and memory. There is the well-known phenomenon of anhedonia in withdrawal, where activities that would normally be pleasurable or rewarding are no longer desirable.

Can you reflect on times when you may have felt anhedonia, and things that would usually be pleasurable felt unappealing or provided no perceived feelings, reward, or relief? Write about what was happening and how that felt.

_____

_____

_____

_____

_____

_____

_____

In a healthy brain, the functions of the cingulate gyrus are:

- *shifting of attention*
- *cognitive flexibility*
- *adaptability*
- *the mind moves from idea to idea*

- *the ability to see options*
- *you go with the flow*
- *cooperation*

Problems in the cingulate gyrus will result in:

- ☐ *worrying or rumination*
- ☐ *holding on to hurts from the past*
- ☐ *stuck on thoughts (obsessions)*
- ☐ *stuck on behaviours (compulsions)*
- ☐ *oppositional behaviour, argumentative*

- ☐ *uncooperative, tendency to say 'no'*
- ☐ *addictive behaviours (alcohol or drug abuse, eating disorders, chronic pain)*
- ☐ *cognitive inflexibility*
- ☐ *obsessive compulsive behaviour*

What symptoms have you experienced from the list above (place a check mark in the appropriate boxes)? When and how have these symptoms impacted your life?

_____

_____

_____

_____

_____

_____

_____

In the questions above, it is important to recognize when you experience symptoms associated with problems in specific areas of your brain as you can then take action to reduce potential triggers or exposure. For example, if you are aware you can have problems with your attention span, procrastination and poor time management when you are feeling stressed, then it is important to take action to reduce or cope with your stress over time. Specific tools will be discussed later in the workbook; for now the focus is to increase awareness of your strengths and vulnerabilities.

As already mentioned, behaviours/characteristics are symptoms of brain health. With Addiction, common behavioural patterns include being compulsive, impulsive, sad, anxious or any combination thereof. The more awareness you have about your behavioural tendencies or vulnerabilities, the more you will understand how Addiction manifests in your life. The following list has been adapted from the work of Dr. Dan Amen.

Using the examples below, which behaviours or characteristics do you commonly experience?
Check all that apply.

1. Compulsive characteristics – flexible thinking challenges

   ☐ *Excessive worrying*
   ☐ *Rigid, want things a certain way*
   ☐ *Get stuck on the same thought over and over*
   ☐ *Hold grudges*
   ☐ *Upset when things do not go a certain way*
   ☐ *Argumentative or oppositional*
   ☐ *Nighttime eater to calm worries*
   ☐ *Compulsive eating behaviour*

2. Impulsive characteristics – difficulty with impulse control

   ☐ *Tendency to speak without thinking, blurt out answers*
   ☐ *Trouble sustaining focus or attention*
   ☐ *Become easily distracted or off task*
   ☐ *Difficulty delaying what you want*
   ☐ *Restless, trouble sitting still*
   ☐ *Impulsively order food later wish hadn't*
   ☐ *Disorganization*
   ☐ *Often late or in a hurry*
   ☐ *Need caffeine for energy or focus*

3. Sad

   ☐ *History of feeling depressed*
   ☐ *Often feel sad*
   ☐ *Negative thinking and self-talk*
   ☐ *Low energy*
   ☐ *Feel joyless*
   ☐ *Feel hopeless*
   ☐ *Moody*
   ☐ *Low self-esteem*
   ☐ *Feel alone*
   ☐ *Eat as a way to boost mood*

4. Anxious

   ☐ *Feel stress*
   ☐ *Feel nervous*
   ☐ *Excessive muscle tension (such as headaches or upset stomach)*
   ☐ *Feel panicky inside*
   ☐ *Tend to predict the worst*
   ☐ *Avoid conflict*
   ☐ *Worry about being judged by others*
   ☐ *Lack confidence*
   ☐ *Easily startled*
   ☐ *Eat, drink alcohol, smoke marijuana as a way to soothe anxious feelings*

Total up your check marks in each category. Any category where you have check marks indicates this may be part of your brain type. You can be one type (e.g., Sad type) or any combination of the types (e.g., Compulsive-Impulsive, Compulsive-Sad-Anxious, Compulsive-Impulsive-Sad-Anxious). Once you recognize your brain type, you can take action to get healthier. Some action items to consider are as follows:

- Having structure in your daily activities

- Setting SMART goals (specific, measurable, attainable, relevant and time sensitive)

- Increasing awareness of the automatic thoughts and addictive thinking

- Daily meditation, which helps decrease high blood pressure, lowers levels of anxiety, as well as promote an overall healthier immune system

- Diaphragmatic breathing – slow, deep breathing to balance out your sympathetic and parasympathetic nervous systems, allowing your body to function more optimally. It helps reduce the stress hormones adrenaline and cortisol

- Listening to relaxing music

- Regular exercise at least three times per week for a minimum of 20 minutes

- A balanced diet of high quality protein and high quality carbohydrates

- Fish oil, Green Tea, Tryptophan
- Optimize vitamin D level (to maintain level between 100–150 nmol/L)

Recovery work is rewarding but it can be emotionally challenging as well. At this point, we would encourage you to pause and take 10 minutes to sit quietly with your eyes closed, allowing whatever thoughts and feelings need to come. You can then let them go and fade away, without attachment. Take time to create a loving space for yourself anytime you see the graphic below in the book. This is your reminder to pause and take a break. You can also do that anytime you need to, even if the graphic is not present. Recovery is about listening to yourself. Taking time to sit with feelings and process what is coming up will help you focus more on being in recovery.

Addiction as a Primary, Chronic Brain Disease

Addiction is a primary, chronic brain disease of brain reward, motivation, memory, and related circuitry. Primary means that it is not caused by anything else and chronic means that it is lifelong in nature. Once someone has the disease of Addiction, it does not go away. A common question asked in treatment is, *what caused me to become addicted?* It is important to understand that there are many risk factors, aggravating factors, and vulnerabilities, but no one external factor is the cause, as research has pointed to genetics as the fundamental contributor.

Addiction is a single condition—hence the title, *Addiction is Addiction*—rather than describing 'addictions' such as that involving alcohol as distinct from Addiction involving cocaine or gambling. This is in contrast to other classification systems, where each substance-related or behaviour-related problem is considered to be a separate problem. Addiction is not limited to alcohol and drugs. It can include:

- *Gambling*
- *Food/eating disorders*
- *High risk behaviours (fighting, stunts, fast driving)*
- *Sex (pornography, use of escorts, masturbation, sex outside of a committed relationship)*
- *Love*
- *Relationships*
- *Internet/video games*
- *Technology (Smartphones)*
- *Media*
- *Fantasy*
- *Money*
- *Shopping*
- *Exercise/sports*
- *Work*
- *Caffeine*
- *Nicotine*
- *Prescription medication*

It is also recognized that Addiction is not just a brain disease. Beyond the biological aspect, disease manifestations occur along psychological, social, and spiritual dimensions. A number of people look at the spiritual dimension as part of psychological or social, but the spiritual is fundamentally about the basic values a person has and what gives meaning to a person's life. The values and meaning in life provide a framework for a human being's relationship to themselves, to beyond oneself with others and further with the transcendent aspect of life or existential connection with the rest of the universe.

What gives meaning in your life?

_____
_____
_____
_____
_____

What are your values?

_____
_____
_____
_____
_____

The term disease can be defined as a condition of the living being or of one of its parts that impairs normal functioning. It is typically manifested by distinguishing, characteristic signs and symptoms. With Addiction, the organ that is impacted is the brain. Injuries, disabilities, disorders, syndromes, infections, isolated symptoms, deviant behaviours, and atypical variations of structure and function can sometimes be called a disease, however, it is important to appreciate that complications and behavioural manifestations are not necessarily the disease. For example, infections result from a problem in the immune system that can leave one vulnerable to recurrent episodes; or behaviour problems can be due to some underlying brain dysfunction. Simply put, a disease is a dysfunction somewhere in the body-brain complex that has a recognizable form in terms of symptoms, which the individual experiences, and signs, which others can see. Therefore, it is important for people to have awareness of symptoms and be attentive to signs that are visible to others but may not be so to the affected individual. Diseases not only affect people physically, but also emotionally, mentally, and spiritually, as living with many diseases can alter one's perspective on life and their behaviour. The result or outcome of a disease may be recovery, disability, or death.

"A chronic disease is one that lasts for a long time, usually more than six months."

A chronic disease is one that lasts for a long time, usually more than six months. During that time, it may be constantly present, or it may go into remission and periodically flare-up as a relapse. A chronic disease may be stable, meaning that it does not get any worse, or it may be progressive, meaning that it gets worse over time. Asthma is an example of a chronic disease involving the airways in the lungs. There is no cure for asthma, but once it is properly diagnosed and a treatment plan is in place, individuals are able to manage their condition, and quality of life will improve. Most chronic diseases can be beneficially treated, even if they cannot be permanently cured. Stress is commonly associated with flare-ups of this disease, which is also true of Addiction.

What do you think defines a disease?

_____
_____
_____
_____
_____

How can you now appreciate Addiction being a disease?

_____

_____

_____

_____

_____

What are your doubts about Addiction being a disease?

_____

_____

_____

_____

_____

Some believe that in viewing Addiction as a disease, it abdicates all responsibility for behaviour. All humans need to take responsibility for their behaviour and be accountable for actions, but blaming oneself or someone for a condition that is beyond their control only increases shame. When the person recognizes that they did not choose to behave badly and that their behaviours are secondary to dysfunction in their brain, they can then start to focus on recovery and appreciate that the disease is only a part of them and not defining of their nature. It is important to remember that you did not choose the disease of Addiction, but you can choose recovery.

Write about your feelings and beliefs that acknowledging having a disease removes accountability.

_____

_____

_____

_____

_____

_____

Genetics of Addiction

Research has shown Addiction to be genetically complex, meaning there is not a single gene, but many genes, that play a role in affecting the form that manifests for each individual. Therefore, it is essential for each individual to honestly appreciate their own experience with Addiction in its myriad forms. This is also the reason where one particular manifestation, for example, alcohol-related problems, may remit once the individual stops using alcohol, yet the disease may manifest in other problem behaviours, such as gambling or overeating.

Genetic factors account for approximately 50–60 per cent of the likelihood that an individual will develop Addiction. However, having a genetic predisposition does not mean that it will occur, as environment also plays a significant role and the manifestations can be quite diverse in severity as well. Over the past few decades, a new science called epigenetics has influenced how we view Addiction and many other diseases, and has broadened our understanding of the roles of nature and nurture. At its most basic level, epigenetics is the study of changes in gene activity and how the genome responds to the environment. Stress, exposure to substances, family, culture, and other factors activate chemical switches that regulate how the genes are expressed. In order for genes to express themselves or be switched 'on', environmental factors need to interact with the person's biology, which then affects the extent to which the genetic factors exert their influence.

All humans are vulnerable as the disease of Addiction is endemic genetically in all peoples around the world. In a world that fosters instant gratification and the desire for more, and easy access to mood altering and socially acceptable substances such as alcohol, tobacco, food or marijuana, it is easy to indulge. Internet, gambling, video games, and pornography are more accessible to individuals of all ages, including children, in so many different venues on many platforms, including social media. Cultural factors also may influence self-concept and behaviour, as well as how we interact with others, react to stress, and deal with our feelings in healthy or unhealthy ways. Normalizing dysfunctional behaviour can increase the likelihood of manifestations of Addiction, whereas more honest and supportive family environments foster resilience, which can be protective to some degree.

What are some unhealthy or dysfunctional behaviors you have witnessed in your friends and/or family that are normalized? An example may be that every time Aunt Betty comes over for dinner, she drinks too much and needs to stay over, take a taxi or be driven home. The family shrugs off her behaviour, "that's just Aunt Betty."

_____

_____

_____

_____

_____

_____

_____

In 2012, the American Society of Addiction Medicine (ASAM), the largest professional association in North America for doctors who are interested in prevention, treatment, medical education, research, and public policy advocacy regarding Addiction and related health conditions, approved a definition of Addiction. It was based on extensive review of current scientific work, lessons learned by experienced clinicians, and experts in research and clinical practice.

DEFINITION OF ADDICTION (SHORT VERSION)

The definition of Addiction as outlined by ASAM is as follows:

> *Addiction is a primary, chronic disease of brain reward, motivation, memory and related circuitry. Dysfunction in these circuits leads to characteristic biological, psychological, social and spiritual manifestations. This is reflected in an individual pathologically pursuing reward and/or relief by substance use and other behaviours.*

> *Addiction is characterized by inability to consistently abstain, impairment in behavioural control, craving, diminished recognition of significant problems with one's behaviours and interpersonal relationships, and a dysfunctional emotional response. Like other chronic diseases, Addiction often involves cycles of relapse and remission. Without treatment or engagement in recovery activities, Addiction is progressive and can result in disability or premature death.*

Addiction is characterized by:

A. Inability to consistently **A**bstain,   B. Impairment in **B**ehavioural control,

C. **C**raving or increased hunger for drugs or reward-ing experiences,

D. **D**iminished recognition of significant problems with one's behaviours and interpersonal relationships, and

E. A dysfunctional **E**motional response.

Abstinence. The 'inability to consistently abstain' emphasizes that short periods of abstinence are achievable within a person with Addiction. These periods may deceptively provide reassurance to the affected individual simply because control does not appear to be lost.

Abstinence is defined by ASAM as a process, as follows:

> *Intentional and consistent restraint from the pathological pursuit of reward and/or relief that involves the use of substances and other behaviors. These behaviors may involve, but are not necessarily limited to, gambling, video gaming, spending, compulsive eating, compulsive exercise, or compulsive sexual behaviors.*

Abstinence may be established in some areas and be elusive in others, but it is essential to address abstinence in treatment or recovery stability will be compromised. The continued pursuit of abstinence from all mood-altering substances and restraint from engaging in unhealthy behaviours is critical for health. This involves exploring areas like your relationship with food, sex, and other behaviours and pursuing restraint around the parts that are particularly activating and aggravating to the disease. For example, potato chips may trigger the desire for more in one person with the disease but not in another. What needs to be abstained from becomes more individualized, but recovery for Addiction beyond drugs and alcohol still needs to include the pursuit of restraint in some form. Abstinence is a central component of long-term sobriety, which requires engagement in recovery to optimize wellness.

Recovery beyond abstinence includes:

- *Incorporating a focus on holistic health and whole being*

- *Gaining awareness of and experience living with feelings, appreciating that there are not 'good' or 'bad' feelings. Just because something may feel bad does not mean it is a bad feeling*

- *Putting life into recovery … not recovery into life*

- *A recovery support network*

- *"It works if you work it" that means active involvement, as opposed to waiting for things to happen*

What have been your challenges in pursuing abstinence?

_____
_____
_____
_____
_____

It is a myth that substance use causes Addiction and is what Addiction is. In reality, substance use is the behavioural manifestation of Addiction. It can aggravate the disease (which already existed because it is genetic). These substances will also have additional effects on the body and mind due to the chemicals involved in them. Tolerance and withdrawal can occur in the context of substance use, as well as with behaviours.

"Substance use can aggravate the disease, but it is not the disease and does not cause it."

Tolerance and withdrawal are physiological adaptations caused by the brain adjusting itself to the periodic or regular presence of substances and/or behaviours over time, which are potentially disrupting the internal balance or homeostasis.

We often hear 'I don't have any withdrawal symptoms so I must not be addicted,' or 'I'm addicted as I need more and more (tolerance) and have withdrawal if I do not get enough.' Both of these statements are misleading, as tolerance and withdrawal commonly occur with Addiction, but are not essential components in its diagnosis. Both tolerance and withdrawal occur in response to anything that affects the brain, so it may or may not be connected to Addiction necessarily.

Tolerance occurs when the brain is exposed to a substance or behaviour over time, causing the brain to become less sensitive to the effects of a particular amount or dose, and requiring more to have the same effect the individual may have desired before. This happens because the body and brain are constantly trying to maintain homeostasis or balance by generating a response that is opposite of the response resulting from using substances or engaging in addictive behaviours. Behaviourally, it can manifest in taking more and more risk because the initial thrill is not so thrilling over time.

How has tolerance affected your life?

_____

_____

_____

_____

_____

Withdrawal is symptoms that occur in the presence or even anticipation of the use of an addictive substance or engagement in addictive behaviours. It occurs in many ways to counter the anticipated effects of substance use and/or behaviours in an effort to maintain stability in the body-mind function. The withdrawal that is triggered from memory in the absence of using substances or acting out behaviourally is called Post Acute Withdrawal Syndrome (PAWS). As Addiction is a complex, lifelong disease of the entire self beyond one's physiology, it is important to look beyond tolerance and withdrawal as sole criteria. It is also important to appreciate that the withdrawal response is stored in memory and can be triggered by people, places, and things, which can lead one to relapse.

What withdrawal symptoms have you noticed? When?

_____

_____

_____

_____

_____

What are your triggers for a withdrawal response

People:

_____

_____

_____

_____

_____

Places:

_____

_____

_____

_____

_____

Things:

_____

_____

_____

_____

_____

THE RELAPSE CONTINUUM

The persistent risk or recurrences of relapse after periods of abstinence is another feature of Addiction. This can be triggered by exposure to rewarding substances and behaviours, environmental cues to use, and emotional stressors that trigger heightened activity in brain stress circuits. In treatment, we refer to *people, places, and things* as powerful triggers for relapse as the memory circuitry is activated. Individuals have found how the smell of alcohol, the taste of non-alcoholic beverages that resemble alcoholic beverages, the sound of slot machines, the sight of fast food commercials on TV, and a caressing touch from the opposite sex can all elicit intense memories and feelings that trigger relapse. Typically, the individual is unaware and needs someone external to them (i.e., peer support groups, therapist, sponsor) to identify the risks and triggers for relapse.

The relapse continuum typically occurs in the following order: *Spiritual– Emotional – Cognitive – Social – Behavioural*. Acting out or relapsing physically is usually the last manifestation so it is important to recognize the earlier signs of relapse behaviour to reduce the risk of relapse.

Spiritual relapse can include:

- Spiritual disconnection or lack of meaning in life

- Living in violation of your values (e.g., honesty, integrity)

- Feeling lonely, contributes to anger and frustration against self and the world, puts one in 'victim' mode

- Time spent reflecting, praying, meditating, and connecting with a Higher Power declines. (A Higher Power is sometimes referred to as a power greater than ourselves and is frequently abbreviated to HP)

What are signs of spiritual relapse for you?

_____

_____

_____

_____

_____

Emotional relapse can include:

- Anger outbursts

- Emotional stuffing, avoiding feelings, including happiness and satisfaction

- Feeling anxious, depressed, frustrated

- Day-to-day situations are hard to process, leave an emotional impact that lasts

- Stress or difficulties in dealing with emotions, is one of the three main contributors to relapse (in addition to environment and exposure to addictive substances and addictive behaviours)

What are signs of emotional relapse for you?

_____

_____

_____

_____

_____

Cognitive relapse can include:

- Minimizing

- Rationalizing

- Justifying

- All-or-nothing thinking

- A busy brain, 'crazy thinking', being on the 'hamster wheel'

- Futurizing/catastrophizing, obsessing about 'worst case scenarios'

- Destructive, negative self-talk

What are signs of cognitive relapse for you?

_____

_____

_____

_____

Social relapse can include:

- Isolating

- Associating with using buddies

- Reaching out to comfortable/easy, familiar people rather than healthy/recovery supports

- Increased shame in relationships, which holds one back from connecting authentically and genuinely

What are signs of social relapse for you?

_____

_____

_____

_____

Behavioural relapse can include:

- Using substances

- Using 'de-alcoholized' beer or wine

- Using behaviours to escape, seek relief and/or reward (e.g., gambling, overeating/binging/purging, compulsive shopping, not sticking to healthy boundaries, acting out sexually with infidelity, pornography, paid partners)

- Playing around with boundaries of behaviours, like using masturbation but stopping before orgasm though masturbation has been something you have been pursuing abstinence on

What are signs of behavioural relapse for you?

_____

_____

_____

_____

_____

To maintain abstinence, it is important to recognize your vulnerabilities.

What are your vulnerabilities in each area?

1. *Environment*

_____

_____

_____

_____

_____

2. *Exposure*

_____

_____

_____

_____

3. *Stress*

_____

_____

_____

_____

_____

Impairment in Behavioural Control. Behavioural manifestations and complications of Addiction, primarily due to impaired control can include:

a. Excessive use or engagement in addictive behaviours, at higher frequencies or quantities than intended, often associated with a persistent desire for and unsuccessful attempts at behavioural control;

Example: Alex has been trying to control her drinking by limiting the number of days she goes out with her friends every month; however, she ends up drinking more than planned (6+ drinks instead of planned 1-2) and has trouble saying 'no' when invited out.

Share your own example(s) of excessive use:

_____

_____

_____

_____

_____

_____

b. Excessive time lost in substance use or recovering from the effects of substance use or engagement in addictive behaviours, with significant adverse impact on social and occupational functioning (e.g., the development of inter-personal relationship problems or the neglect of responsibilities at home, school, or work).

Example: Joe has been so busy at work, putting in long hours, which people do not appreciate, as his efficiency is declining and he is making more errors. Further, his wife is upset with him because he is not at home to share in household responsibilities, especially time with children.

Share your own example(s) of excessive time lost due to use of substances or behaviours:

_____

_____

_____

_____

_____

_____

c. Continued use or engagement in addictive behaviours, despite the presence of persistent or recurrent physical or psychological problems, which may have been caused or exacerbated by substance use or related addictive behaviours.

Example: Joan has worsening knee pain because of the extra weight she has put on over the last five years. It is limiting her ability to walk. She has been trying to restrict her food intake yet binging and night-time eating that she cannot control are making her frustrated and depressed.

Share your own example(s) of continued use despite consequences:

_____

_____

_____

_____

_____

_____

d. A narrowing of the behavioural repertoire focusing on rewards that are part of Addiction;

Example: Sam has been spending so much time on online video games, especially at night, that he is losing touch with his regular friends and family.

Share your own example(s) of when and how you left parts of life behind because of other behaviours:

_____

_____

_____

_____

_____

_____

_____

e. An apparent lack of ability or readiness to take consistent, ameliorative action despite recognition of problems.

Example: Bill has noticed that too much money is going into cocaine and gambling, so he has taken to carrying less cash around with him. Yet, ATM machines have become a strong attraction when he runs out of the little cash that he carries.

Share your own example(s) of the challenges you have had with action:

_____

_____

_____

_____

_____

_____

_____

The feature of impairment in behavioural control means engaging in behaviours even when it compromises one's values and beliefs. This is a part of the disease that friends, family members, and colleagues have a difficult time appreciating, as often they believe that the hurtful words, lying, and acting out are intentional and meant to cause pain. The person with Addiction is impaired and not in control of their actions when the disease is active. It is very important to not shame or blame the person for what has been happening. People with Addiction are internally upset already and magnifying that only pushes the shame deeper into darkness, where it festers and grows. Accountability is better enforced by boundaries and consequences. For example, not being around someone who has alcohol-related problems and is still drinking; or not having dinner with someone who is spending more time on their phone than being present at the dinner table. Responsibility and accountability can also be around recovery action to talk about what recovery means and how the individual is progressing rather than failing

Expecting a person with Addiction to control their behaviour is illogical, as the 'B' characteristic of the disease illustrates with impairment in behavioural control. Since the disease is always present, there will be periodic struggles with maintaining consistent abstinence and impaired behavioural control will pop up periodically, which is why accountability over recovery action is needed, not blaming, shaming, or expectations around trying to control the disease.

List three things to help you become more responsible and accountable for your recovery action:

1.

2.

3.

Craving. The subjective experience of craving is impactful to people who have Addiction and it can be a major driving force in relapse. Individuals may experience craving as emotional, cognitive, or physiological, and the behavioural outflows of craving can be experienced as obsession, compulsion, or impulsive behaviour, which may occur seemingly inexplicably to the person. If the craving is satisfied in some other form than the original problem substance or behaviour, the person may even insist that they do not have craving or impairment in behavioural control.

Example: Adam's long-term girlfriend just broke up with him. He cannot stop thinking about her. He ends up driving past her house to see if she is home, checking her social media several times a day. When asked, he says that he is doing well as he has not had any contact with her.

Write about how you have experienced cravings in the past.

_____

_____

_____

_____

_____

Craving describes the need to fulfill an obsessive desire. Craving is a part of the human condition and our brains are hardwired to appreciate and pursue pleasurable and natural rewards such as food and sex because of their survival value. When someone craves something and the desire is fulfilled, dopamine levels in the brain increase. Dopamine is a neurotransmitter that helps control the brain's reward and pleasure centres. It sends signals to the brain that tell us something feels good, which makes us want to do it again. In Addiction, the brain is wired to seek and/or tolerate more dopamine and there is no shutoff valve to say enough, so the individual wants more. When the reward circuits are activated, cravings for alcohol, drugs, or addictive behaviours become increasingly intense, seeking a way to get more dopamine, which may be inherently low due to the genetics or depleted due to excessive demand on the circuits over time.

Dealing with cravings is the responsibility of the brain's inhibitory circuit, which in the healthy brain leads to *stop*, *no more* or *enough*. With Addiction, this inhibitory circuit is dysfunctional so the Addiction brain leads an individual to the opposite signal, which is *go* or *more*. The cravings intensify until the person with Addiction acts out with that substance or behaviour and gets relief, however brief.

How have you dealt with cravings?

_____
_____
_____
_____
_____

How effective has this been?

_____
_____
_____
_____
_____

The power of external cues to trigger cravings typically begins outside our conscious awareness as our brain responds to cues as brief as thirty-three milliseconds, which can activate the reward circuitry and subsequent acting out with substance or behaviour. One may not have conscious awareness of what the trigger or activator was, even though the effects of activation may become overwhelming. For example, walking down the street and seeing a park bench. This seems innocuous but may be associated with going for walks with a loved one who has ended the relationship. The person then experiences thoughts about this person, even though they have not thought about them in months.

Helping an individual appreciate the cues or triggers that lead them to relapse can be challenging, as it is typically not in their conscious awareness. Cravings can be viewed as intense memories. Brain imaging studies have shown brain activation when pictures that are linked to drug use (like a pipe or a white powdery substance resembling cocaine) are shown to people who have Addiction. These memories are the brain re-experiencing an event, so reliving a drug, sex, or other past compulsive experience can cause a serious emotional reaction. This is the reason why romantic notions (thoughts or feelings) connected with any aspect of Addiction trigger craving. For instance, carrying feelings of joy or happiness associated with drugs, alcohol, food, people, sexual experiences, gambling or more. Let us take the time to explore the romantic notions you are still carrying about particular substances and behaviours.

What beliefs do you carry about the value and benefit of alcohol?

_____
_____
_____
_____
_____

What beliefs do you carry about the value and benefit of drugs (cocaine, marijuana, prescription medication, heroin, opioids, LSD, hallucinogens, etc.)?

_____
_____
_____

_____
_____

Caffeine?

_____
_____
_____
_____
_____

Sex, love, and relationships?

_____
_____
_____
_____
_____

Gambling?

_____
_____
_____
_____
_____
_____

Food?

_____
_____
_____
_____
_____

Media and technology (e.g., iPads, Smartphones, Internet)?

_____
_____
_____
_____
_____

When compulsive thought revolves around a desire, then craving and ritualized behaviour often follows. For example, not being able to stop thinking about going online and using pornography will lead to craving to act out, which can result in this behaviour happening. With cravings, brain areas associated with the sights, sounds, smells, and thoughts related to the event are activated in a manner similar to the initial experience. Cravings can be triggered by any of the five senses. This is why it is important to minimize exposure to substances, as well as environments and people that increase vulnerability. The worst thing someone in recovery can do is test themselves by going into dangerous situations to prove the strength of their recovery. As we have been discussing, the brain never loses its vulnerability for this disease and can be activated quickly, even if the intention is to be in recovery. For example, going to pubs repeatedly while not drinking and others around you are, thinking that this is healthy and must mean your recovery is strong. Meanwhile, with repeated exposure there is likely to be an increase in compulsive thoughts, craving, and ritualized behaviour. In other words, the more exposure, the more likely it is that someone will find themselves relapsing. People in recovery circles have sometimes referred to cravings as 'obsession of the mind', which can turn into 'allergy of the body'– compulsion or impaired control over behaviours, despite the individual's best intentions not to engage in them.

When and how have you tested out your recovery strength?

_____
_____
_____
_____
_____

How did you feel after these tests?

_____
_____
_____
_____
_____

What does 'obsession of the mind' mean to you?

_____
_____
_____
_____
_____

What does 'allergy of the body' mean to you?

_____
_____
_____
_____
_____

Cravings can be experienced physically but they can also be felt psychologically and come into people's dreams, with 'using dreams' being a very common experience for people in recovery, even long-term. Rather than panic about these experiences, it is important to view them as valuable information. Your brain is trying to tell you something about your vulnerability that needs to be addressed. There is a lot of opportunity in these experiences and they provide helpful reminders to be consistently diligent in one's health and recovery.

Have you ever had using dreams? Write down the dreams here and what they signified to you.

_____
_____
_____

_____
_____

What information was provided by that dream/those dreams?

_____
_____
_____
_____
_____

While cravings may seem to come randomly at times, there is a lot of information that we can learn from them. It is important to remember cravings are a symptom and consequence of the disease, not a reflection of recovery knowledge or strength.

> *"It is important to remember cravings are a symptom and consequence of the disease, not a reflection of recovery knowledge or strength."*

The additional two characteristics of the disease, the 'D' and 'E' are discussed next.

Diminished recognition of significant problems with one's behaviours and interpersonal relationships. In Addiction, there is significant impairment in executive functioning, which manifests in problems with perception, learning, impulse control, compulsivity, and judgement. People with Addiction often manifest a lower readiness to change their dysfunctional behaviours despite mounting concerns expressed by significant others in their lives. They display an apparent lack of appreciation of the magnitude of cumulative problems and complications. They may keep drinking, using drugs, gambling, spending, using sex for escape, and staying in abusive and unhealthy relationships despite it being apparent to those around them that these behaviours are killing them.

The profound drive to use substances or engage in apparently rewarding behaviours, with or without craving, with apparent disregard to adverse consequences that is seen in most people with Addiction, underscores the compulsive aspect of this disease. This is the correlation with "powerlessness" over Addiction and "unmanageability" of life, as is described in Step 1 of 12-Step programs.

Many blind spots exist in the disease of Addiction and characteristic 'D' highlights that they exist with behaviour and relationships. This is the fundamental reason why external support is a necessary part of the recovery process to reduce problems in behaviour and relationships that are not visible to the person with Addiction. It is hard for the person with Addiction to see clearly what is happening in their relationships and life, as things are being filtered through the disease and become skewed. While the A, B, and C characteristics tend to diminish significantly in the context of abstinence and recovery, the D and E characteristics are the lifelong aspects of Addiction. While behaviours such as food, relationships, sex, work, exercise, and shopping cannot be completely abstained from, it is important to be aware that there is still a necessary abstinence component to these behaviours in the context of recovery. In behaviours beyond drugs and alcohol, it is more individualized what specific parts of the behaviour the person will need to abstain from. For example, not going into bakeries or fast food restaurants for one person may be an essential part of their recovery, whereas for another it is prioritizing not having chips, crackers, or pasta in their home. For individuals pursuing recovery with behaviours beyond drugs and alcohol, the pursuit of abstinence from drugs and alcohol is also a necessary component to recovery and health in addition to the pursuit of restraint from other activities, environments, or behaviours.

Checking in with the people in your life for their perspective is an important part of not getting trapped in 'D'. It is recommended that these people be in recovery themselves and/or have familiarity with what Addiction is and the language of recovery.

Identify your main supports in recovery that you can "check in" or "check it out" with?

1.

2.

3.

4.

Are these supports in recovery themselves? What is their understanding of Addiction from what you can gather?

_____
_____
_____
_____
_____

It is important to process the specifics of situations with people in recovery or those who understand recovery so that they can provide feedback and highlight any disease activity they can see that the person with Addiction cannot.

How often do you check in with or check things out with others in recovery?

_____
_____
_____

What challenges do you find with checking in or checking things out?

_____
_____
_____
_____
_____

What benefits do you find with checking in or checking things out?

_____
_____
_____

_____

_____

Can you challenge yourself to check in with other people and check things out more consistently?

We would recommend having a conversation with somebody in recovery every day in order to increase comfort with being open and vulnerable, as well as consistent practice in getting feedback. There can be a lot of disease activity within a 24-hour period.

Dysfunctional Emotional response. Emotional changes with Addiction can include:

a. Increased anxiety, dysphoria, (feeling unwell or unhappy) and emotional pain. This may alternate with feelings of mania, stimulation, or euphoria (feeling invincible, giddy)

b. Increased sensitivity to stressors associated with the recruitment of brain stress systems, such that "things seem more stressful" as a result

c. Difficulty in identifying feelings, distinguishing between feelings and the bodily sensations of emotional arousal, and describing feelings to other people (sometimes referred to as alexithymia).

Which of the symptoms above have you experienced? Write more about these experiences and how they felt at the time.

_____

_____

_____

_____

_____

_____

_____

Emotion arises at the place where mind and body meet; it is part of the body's reaction to the mind. If there is a conflict between thought and emotion, the thought will be the lie (often created by the disease) and the emotion will be the relative truth about how you feel at that time, even if coloured by dysfunction. It is essential not to judge our feelings or thoughts; rather, we need to pay attention to them. For example, you may understand that your parent was unwell when they ignored you and were emotionally unavailable, but this does not erase the feelings of sadness, anger, resentment, and shame that are present.

The dysfunctional emotional response is one of the lifelong components of the disease and characteristics include:

- Making a molehill out of a mountain (minimization, under or no reaction)

- Making a mountain out of a molehill (exaggeration, strong or over reaction)

- All-or-nothing response (otherwise known as black and white thinking)

- Numbing, avoiding, escaping feelings

- Emotional language may be missing

- Unaware of emotions that are there
- Taking on other people's feelings as your own

The dysfunctional emotional response often manifests in OUTBURSTS and/or STUFFING of emotions and contributes to difficulties in relationships.

What are your responses to emotional situations? List some examples here.

_____
_____
_____
_____
_____

What difficulties have these responses created in your relationships?

_____
_____
_____
_____
_____

The Volcano Effect

When feelings are not communicated and dealt with, they can boil beneath the surface and eventually cause so much pressure that they erupt like a volcano.

Can you give some examples of when you have erupted?

1.

2.

3.

What feelings can you identify that you were stuffing or suppressing in each example?

1.

2.

3.

The two most common concerns for people living with someone with Addiction are: 1) substance use or problem behaviours and 2) issues with feelings. The emotional challenges can include: anger outbursts, suicidal ideation, over reaction, under reaction, being numb and cold, and emotional unpredictability. Many people believe that these feelings-based challenges are the direct result of the substance use or problematic behaviours and believe that if the person would just stop using, that they would become emotionally healthy. This is not the case.

Emotional health in the context of Addiction is a major component of the recovery work that is needed and takes time and effort to explore and develop. Identification of, connection with, and healthy expression of feelings does not come easily or naturally to people with Addiction and takes time, patience and understanding from everybody. Feelings are a major driver of this disease and need to be regarded with the importance they carry, without falling into the trap that emotional dysfunction is all down to the brain being high or intoxicated. In reality, emotional dysfunction is the second lifelong, persistent part of the disease in addition to diminished recognition of problems in relationships and behaviours and, as such, needs to be discussed and explored, not feared. Feelings do not kill us; they provide valuable information, but will kill the person with Addiction, sometimes by suicide, if they continue to be numbed and avoided.

Let us practice doing an emotional check-in. Stop, close your eyes for a few moments and ask yourself "how have I been feeling today?" List as many feelings as you can, no matter how seemingly insignificant or contradictory.

_____

_____

_____

_____

_____

_____

As emotional health is an integral part of recovery, we encourage you to check-in on your feelings at least once daily in order to keep improving the quality and depth of your relationship with your feelings (and self).

ADDICTION, MENTAL HEALTH, AND PSYCHIATRIC DISORDERS

Mental health problems are common and occur in all of us. We all feel sad, mad, or bad from time to time. We have different coping styles, based on our experience and our environment, to deal with whatever is going on that is unpleasant. Addiction as a brain disease creates a vulnerability in which mental health problems are either ignored, avoided, or magnified, especially in terms of blaming other people, places, or things rather than taking personal responsibility. Feelings are often repressed and suppressed such that they commonly come out in the form of anxiety and depression.

Do you view anxiety and depression as independent mental health issues from Addiction or symptoms of Addiction? Write about where this belief and understanding comes from.

_____

_____

_____

_____

_____

Anxiety is a very common symptom of Addiction and many people struggle with anxiety long before they act out with substances or behaviours in an effort to numb and seek relief. Anxiety-related problems are fear-based. The fear is usually of things in the future that may or may not happen, yet the person experiences them as not just a possibility but as if they were happening right then, thus creating an overwhelming emotional response that the individual wants to escape. They may recognize the fear is totally unrealistic, but this does not make the feeling less real. Once in active Addiction, fear and anxiety become magnified when someone does not know how or when they will get their next hit of the drug, in addition to anxiety being a common withdrawal reaction that physiologically results in more drug seeking. Panic attacks are an extreme example that can happen in the context of alcohol and drug use, or during withdrawal.

Symptoms of anxiety commonly include (check all that have applied to you):

☐ *Feelings of panic, fear, and uneasiness*
☐ *Problems sleeping*
☐ *Cold or sweaty hands or feet*
☐ *Shortness of breath*
☐ *Heart palpitations*
☐ *Not being able to be still and calm*

☐ *Dry mouth*
☐ *Numbness or tingling in the hands or feet*
☐ *Nausea*
☐ *Digestive issues (e.g., diarrhea)*
☐ *Dizziness, feeling lightheaded or faint*
☐ *Muscle tension*

What words would you use to describe your anxiety?

_____
_____
_____
_____
_____

Would you describe yourself as a highly anxious, moderately anxious, or a rarely anxious person? What does that mean and look like for you?

_____
_____
_____
_____
_____

How do you experience the feeling of anxiety in your body, mind, and emotions?

_____
_____
_____
_____
_____

What you do to manage anxiety when you feel it?

_____
_____
_____
_____
_____

How have your responses to these questions changed over time? What does this tell you about your relationship with anxiety and fear?

_____
_____
_____

_____
_____

As already mentioned, anxiety-related problems are fear-based. Fear will keep you paralyzed as it is difficult to change when we are worried about 'what if'. Faith is the complete trust or confidence in someone or something and an antidote to FEAR (False Evidence Appearing Real). Faith allows us to move through our lives freely, believing that things will work out as they need, not as we may think they *should*. For example, rather than believing that you should be able to pick up a musical instrument and be proficient at it, you trust that with time, practice, and experience the process will unfold as it needs to. Perhaps you are not musically-minded and you can be accepting of that.

Write down some examples of False Evidence Appearing Real that you have experienced:

_____
_____
_____
_____
_____
_____

Depression is also a common withdrawal symptom connected to all aspects of Addiction, both chemical and behavioural. It is a reflection of the distress experienced when one cannot get what one desires, is losing what one desires, or realizes that what was once pleasurable is no longer so. It reflects the increasing recognition that one is at a place where one did not want to be. Depression is usually associated with regret, guilt, and shame, which in thinking escalates from 'I shouldn't have done that' to 'I did bad' to 'I am bad.' The chemical imbalance that results in the brain related to depression may require anti-depressant treatment; however, these medications are quite ineffective if one remains in active Addiction with or without ongoing alcohol or drug use.

Depression is not …

Most times when you feel down, you are not depressed. Feeling sad or low is a big part of life and cannot be avoided. When something goes wrong in your life, whether it is an argument with your partner, conflict with your boss, or a physical illness, your mood might drop. If you feel especially sad or irritable because of this situation, maybe with poor sleep, not wanting to see friends or family, eating too much or not enough, then you are probably experiencing low mood. Low mood will typically go away in a week or two, especially if there is an improvement in the situation that activated it.

Depression is …

1. *If your mood is very low or you have almost no interest in your life almost every day, and this feeling goes on for weeks AND*

2. *If you have other problems like (check all that apply to you):*

   ☐ *big changes in weight or appetite;*
   ☐ *not being able to sleep enough or sleeping too much;*
   ☐ *feeling that you are always restless or slowed-down;*
   ☐ *thinking that you are worthless or useless;*

☐ *feeling really tired much of the time;*
☐ *feeling numb or empty;*
☐ *having a lot of trouble concentrating or making decisions;*
☐ *thinking about death or suicide;*
☐ *attempting or planning suicide or other escape.*

It is important to gain understanding and awareness around the feelings that may contribute to depression, specifically regret (sad about missed opportunities), guilt (upset about things we have done/not done), and shame (feeling overall less than and unworthy, sometimes for no apparent reason or cause).

What do I regret?

_____

_____

_____

_____

_____

What do I feel guilty about?

_____

_____

_____

_____

_____

When do I feel shame?

_____

_____

_____

_____

_____

Anxiety and depression symptoms can vary from mild to severe. It is crucial for people to seek help if the symptoms are persisting or getting worse. When someone has Addiction, the prognosis is promising if these are a complication of Addiction because the symptoms that led to these diagnoses often remit once Addiction is treated effectively and the individual maintains ongoing recovery.

Psychiatric diagnoses such as attention deficit disorder (ADD), attention deficit hyperactivity disorder (ADHD), bipolar disorder (BD) and borderline personality disorder (BPD) are also part of Addiction, rather than separate entities that they are made out to be by some professionals. More severe mental illness, such as schizophrenia or psychoses, can occur concurrently with Addiction, thus requiring more intensive and specialized treatment with medication. In these situations, proper medications, close monitoring, and continuing care are critical to maintaining a healthy recovery.

What psychiatric diagnoses have you received in the past?

_____

_____

_____

_____

What medications have you been given in the past or are taking currently to deal with the symptoms?

_____

_____

_____
_____

What and how do you feel about the connections made in this section between Addiction and Mental Health problems?

_____
_____
_____
_____

TRAUMA

The human brain function is dependent on the physical, chemical, and emotional environment, such that it can go into dysfunction acutely or chronically when exposed to trauma. This can include physical trauma like brain injury, chemical trauma like exposure to substances, and emotional trauma like physical, emotional, or sexual abuse. The vulnerability is even greater during fetal development in pregnancy and early childhood development, from birth to age six. Age seven to sixteen is a period of rapid learning and development that can be hampered by trauma. The vulnerability continues between ages seventeen and twenty-five as well, in terms of executive functioning, decision-making, and becoming responsible. Risk-taking behaviours that are common during late adolescence and early adult life are part of growing up, yet create a vulnerability to all forms of trauma and can hamper further development.

"Trauma is a strong aggravating factor for Addiction and must be dealt with within the framework of recovery."

Some people erroneously believe that trauma is the cause of Addiction, as they search for a reason why someone may be using substances or engaging in addictive behaviours. The reality is that not everyone who experiences trauma goes on to suffer from Addiction, and many people with Addiction have had no trauma prior to their disease becoming manifest. However, trauma is a strong aggravating factor and must be dealt with within the framework of recovery. Some stability is needed with recovery structure, as trauma therapy without that leads to more emotional pain, thus increasing the desire to escape, which makes the Addiction worse.

It is the genetic predisposition, combined with a host of environmental issues, that determines when and how the disease of Addiction becomes manifest, gets complicated, and can ultimately be fatal if left untreated or is poorly treated. Poor treatment can include just focusing on substance use, ignoring underlying emotional, spiritual and mental health vulnerabilities, and/or introducing medications that are contraindicated for people with Addiction.

What has been your understanding about the link between trauma and Addiction?

_____
_____
_____
_____
_____

How has this served your recovery?

_____
_____
_____
_____
_____

How has this inhibited your recovery?

_____
_____
_____
_____
_____

Post-traumatic stress disorder (PTSD) is a specific psychiatric disorder that is often present in people with Addiction. When one appreciates the brain vulnerability, it is easy to understand that someone who has manifest Addiction or a high degree of genetic predisposition would be more prone to PTSD. The inability to deal with feelings in a healthy manner creates conditions in the brain in which repeated flashbacks can be triggered. Intrusive memories represent interference by the past with present brain function and can lead to erratic behaviour, aggression, nightmares, and sleep dysfunction. Commonly prescribed pain medications or anti-anxiety medications that may provide initial quick relief, ultimately, make Addiction-related problems worse. Treating PTSD as a separate entity does not make Addiction go away. Rather, treating Addiction makes PTSD treatment more effective, largely because there is considerable overlap between the effective treatment approaches, such as individual and group psychotherapy for dealing with painful memories and feelings in general, for both conditions.

What trauma have you experienced in your life?

_____
_____
_____
_____
_____

What thoughts or feelings persist from those events or memories?

_____
_____
_____
_____
_____

How much are you caught in blaming someone or something for the trauma? Write about this here (thoughts, feelings, beliefs):

_____
_____
_____
_____
_____
_____
_____

How much do you blame yourself for the trauma? Write about this here (thoughts, feelings, beliefs):

_____

_____

_____

_____

_____

_____

It is crucial to explore trauma from the perspective of it being an aggravator for the disease, not the cause. The feelings that came from the trauma will need to be processed in order for recovery to progress, but this is not the final phase of recovery and needs to be included as part of the holistic recovery process. It is important to start processing the trauma and doing trauma-specific counselling only once a foundation in abstinence and recovery has been established, otherwise exploring the traumatic event(s) can be very destabilizing and promote a resurgence in addictive behaviour.

Key messages

- The brain is the organ of judgement, personality, character, and decision making. Our behaviour is a result of brain function.

- With Addiction, behaviours are not the disease, nor do they cause it.

- The term 'disease' broadly refers to a dysfunctional state or an abnormal condition that affects one or more organs. With Addiction, that organ is the brain.

- Addiction as a primary, chronic brain disease of brain reward, motivation, memory, and related circuitry requires clarity in understanding that primary means that it is not caused by anything else; and chronic means that it is lifelong in its myriad manifestations.

- Mental health problems are common and occur in all of us. Addiction as a brain disease, however, creates vulnerabilities such that mental health problems are ignored, avoided, or magnified. Feelings are often repressed and suppressed such that they commonly come out in the form of anxiety and depression.

- Trauma is not the cause of Addiction but it is definitely a strong aggravating factor and must be dealt with in the framework of recovery. Some stability is needed with recovery structure, as trauma therapy without that leads to more emotional pain, thus increasing the desire to escape, which makes Addiction worse.

Action steps for Chapter 2 (follow through after chapter exercises)

In this chapter you were exposed to more about Addiction as a primary, chronic brain disease. This may run counter to you and your support network's opinions about Addiction. Moving forward, it would be important to continue your exploration of Addiction by continuing to learn more from others around you as well as resources. We recommend using the Resources for Further Learning section in the back of the book as a starting point for additional information.

Chapter 3: Addictive Thinking

"The world as we have created it is a process of our thinking. It cannot be changed without changing our thinking."
—Albert Einstein

Addictive thinking is a key feature of the disease and involves distortion, abnormal thinking, obsession, and often attempts to control things that cannot be controlled. Addictive thinking is a way for the disease to trap the individual into unhealthy and dysfunctional thought patterns that can seem very seductive and logical, but inherently are illogical and dangerous. For example, that behaviours are not as out of control as they are; that doing cocaine would be a helpful way to deal with an eating issue because you have not had an issue with cocaine in the past; that everyone in the room is looking at you and judging you; or that you are an unworthy and useless person who has little to offer others.

"An interesting characteristic of addictive thinking is that it can be impossible to see in oneself, but can be very easy to see in other people."

Seeing problems in thinking in other people can be an opportunity to consider if there may be problems in one's own thinking. This is the reason that having a network of people who understand Addiction and recovery is so important. Their feedback, as well as your reactions, can provide lots of information.

What traits, behaviours, or statements have you seen or heard recently in others that have created a reaction in you?

_____
_____
_____
_____
_____

What can these reactions tell you about yourself?

_____
_____
_____
_____
_____

Stay in process as you learn what these reactions to others may be informing you of in yourself. For example, if you perceive someone is being selfish and only thinking of themselves and you feel angry about this, you likely feel shame that you have been selfish in the past and/or you carry fear about acting this way yourself. If you are reacting to the issue in someone else; this is often an issue that you are carrying.

"If you spot it, you've got it."

Characteristics of Addictive Thinking

1. *It is Irrational*

   - *Addictive thinking is illogical, unreasonable, and irrational*

   - *It can make sense on the surface but, when examined, does not*

Example: "I cannot take any time off work right now as I have no one to replace me. Cocaine gives me more energy, helps me stay awake so I can work longer hours to get my job done. Once I find someone to replace me, I will cut back on my use, maybe even consider treatment but for now work and cocaine have to go hand in hand."

Please write down some examples of irrational thinking and behaviour (personal or observed).

_____

_____

_____

_____

_____

2. *It is contradictory*

   - *The message changes from moment to moment*

Examples:
"I want to get help ... Things are fine, there is no need for change."

"I can see how hurtful that relationship was for me ... I wish they would text me or reach out to me."

"It's been three weeks since I watched pornography and I feel great, but it would feel relieving to watch some."

Please write down some examples of contradictions (personal or observed).

_____

_____

_____

_____

_____

Rationalization, denial, projection, and minimization are all defence mechanisms or psychological strategies that take place by the unconscious mind to manipulate, deny, or distort reality to maintain a socially acceptable self-image. Healthy people typically use different defences throughout life as coping mechanisms to reduce anxiety generated by various threats, but with active Addiction, these defence mechanisms become significantly heightened.

3. *Rationalization*

   - *Not to be confused with 'irrationality'*

   - *Rationalizations are reasons/excuses for behaviours, they are 'rational lies'*

   - *The mind of the person with Addiction backtracks: it acts first (automatically, quickly) then tries to fill in the blank of "why would I have done that?"*

Example: "I have to see my ex-wife at least once a week as we share custody of our dog. I find this very stressful and don't like seeing her but I have no other option right now."

Please write down some examples of the last time you or someone you know was rationalizing.

_____
_____
_____
_____
_____

4. Minimization

- Often goes hand-in-hand with rationalization
- It lessens the perceived consequences of Addiction, including the impact on self and others
- Form of avoidance and feeds into denial
- "Things aren't so bad"
- "What's the big deal? I'm fine"

Example: "I'm fine with my husband and sons drinking beer around me. Even though they often get out of hand, I never liked beer so it doesn't bother me."

Please write down some examples of minimization in yourself or someone you know.

_____
_____
_____
_____
_____

5. Denial

- The part of the brain with Addiction sends messages that everything is okay, though reality may be quite different
- Is a defence mechanism to protect the Addiction
- Often this is an unconscious process
- Denial sparks anger and frustration from others: "Can't they see what this is doing to him/her/us?"
- The struggling person with Addiction may want to change and see consequences, but is overwhelmed by and entrenched in the disease

Example: "My sister and mother seem overly concerned about my marijuana use and think I've become antisocial. I don't see the problem as it helps me relax and take a break, as I need time for myself."

Please write down some examples of denial in yourself or someone you know.

_____
_____
_____
_____
_____

6. *Avoidance*

- *People believe they are lazy or procrastinators, when really the underlying process is avoidance, or escape*

- *Often fear is involved that fuels the addictive mind's need to avoid*

- *Not wanting to hurt someone else's feelings or spark conflict*

- *Pretending things are not bothering you to protect someone else*

- *Going out of your way to not run into someone who is concerned about you or wants to talk*

Example: "I'm really frustrated with my best friend right now but don't want to rock the boat so I am ignoring her calls this week."

Please write down some examples of avoidance in yourself or someone you know.

_____
_____
_____
_____
_____

7. *All-or-Nothing*

- *Addictive Thinking does not live in the 'grey zone', it is black or white*

- *Remember Addiction is a disease of MORE; therefore it's ALL or it's not happening!*

- *If perfection cannot be achieved, no attempts will be made at change*

- *Easy to focus on what's not happening or not working with all-or-nothing thinking, become disconnected from recovery*

Example: "I was training for a half marathon race but don't feel ready for it. My father suggested I run the 10km instead but I'm not okay with that. I've decided to not enter the race at all."

Please write down some examples of all-or-nothing thinking in yourself or someone you know.

_____
_____
_____
_____
_____

8. *Morbid Expectations*

- *Anticipating the worst will happen*

- *Catastrophizing*

- *Can lead to hypervigilance – always planning for the worst possible outcome and thinking up ways to control the situation and prevent this outcome from happening*

- *Substances can fuel paranoia*

- *Can be paralyzing*

- *Even when things are going well, people with Addiction have a tendency to feel burdened by morbid expectations and their brain may sabotage the situation because they feel undeserving of things going well.*

Example: "My daughter keeps asking me to let her get her driver's licence. I'm so afraid she might get in a car accident once she starts driving that I cannot give my consent."

Many people with Addiction will describe themselves as 'self-sabotaging' and say that they 'give in' to their disease, which is not an accurate description of reality. Rather, Addiction leads them to a destructive outcome with or without their conscious awareness. Thus, it is not the person that is purposefully out to sabotage a situation, but rather it is a consequence of their disease. Sometimes this happens before the person is aware; it is not that they have chosen to 'give in' to something.

Please write down some examples of morbid expectations that you have experienced.

_____

_____

_____

_____

_____

9. *Skewed Time*

- *Addiction is a brain disease impacting memory circuitry, which affects perception of time*

- *Periods of abstinence – hours, days, a few weeks – may 'prove' to the person with Addiction that this is possible 'any time' when in reality, this is not the case*

- *"I have been abstinent for a while now" – reality is two days. Be specific!*

Example: "It feels like ages since I last ate compulsively but when I checked my journal, it had only been 10 days. I thought it had been at least a month!"

Please write down some examples of skewed time that you have experienced.

_____

_____

_____

_____

_____

*To deal with this, it is important to take recovery one day, hour, **or** minute at a time:*

- *"One moment at a time"*

- *Try to focus on the here and now, not get distracted by:*

    The past → *the predominant feeling is Shame (depression)*

    The future → *the predominant feeling is Fear (anxiety)*

- *The present can come with lots of feelings, but these will pass*

- *"Time takes time"*

How do you practice living one moment at a time? If you are not doing this now, how could you incorporate it?

_____
_____
_____
_____
_____

10. *Guilt and Shame*

- *Addictive thinking changes guilt into shame*

- *Rather than think "I did bad" the person with Addiction personalizes these events as "I am bad"*

- *Can make the person with Addiction feel that getting well is futile*

- *12-Step Programs and recovery can help transform shame back into guilt through fearless personal inventory, sharing with others, and making amends*

Example: "It's my fault that my mother is mad at me, I should have been more thoughtful and a better daughter."

Please write down some examples of your behaviours that you feel guilty about.

_____
_____
_____
_____
_____

Please write down some examples of shame that you experience connected with people, places or things.

_____
_____
_____
_____
_____

11.Hypersensitivity, sometimes called reactivity

- *Shame filters experiences in such a way the mind of the person with Addiction takes it personally (e.g., everyone is staring at me, my friend isn't calling because they know I have Addiction, I was declined the promotion because I'm a bad performer)*

- *The 'E' in the ASAM definition: Dysfunctional Emotional Response (exaggerated response to events)*

- *Ego/grandiosity of the disease fuels belief "It's all about me"*

Example: "I don't like sharing my story with a bunch of strangers at meetings. I hate when everyone is staring at me. It feels like they are all judging me."

Please write down some examples of hypersensitivity or reactivity in yourself.

_____

_____

_____

_____

_____

12.Illusion of Control

- *Belief that "I can do it on my own"*

- *Leads to people drinking again after years of sobriety eg., "I can keep it at one this time"*

- *"I know best"*

- *Addiction is unmanageable and you are powerless*

- *Control is a trap laid out by Addiction*

- *Control disconnects people from disease concept – belief that "I just need to try harder"*

- *Isolates people*

- *Builds shame, wondering why you cannot 'succeed' although you are an intelligent person*

Example: "I just need to not get angry anymore then I won't need a drink to calm down."

Please write down some examples of illusion of control.

_____

_____

_____

_____

_____

The feeling of being in charge, of having a say over what happens in one's life, is beneficial for the achievement of life goals. Having self-confidence is about discipline and personal accountability. It must not be confused with control related to addictive thinking. Everyone falls somewhere along the continuum of control and it is a bigger issue for some, while not so much for others. For many people, control can be an issue that gets in the way, especially in the most critical aspects of life. With Addiction, the desire for control goes awry and becomes a trap. The inability to admit impairment in control or inability to control everything, which is often seen as manipulation by others, is characteristic of addictive thinking. With Addiction, the illusion of control must first be addressed for a person in recovery to admit and accept powerlessness over their disease. It is essential to acknowledge the power of Addiction to be able to surrender and discover personal power through recovery.

What parts of your thinking, feeling, and behaviour do you have control over?

_____

_____

_____

_____

_____

What parts of your thinking, feeling, and behaviour do you not have control over?

_____

_____

_____

_____

_____

There are many reasons that lead us to control. People's beliefs and feelings lead them to control others, certain situations, money, communication, food, workflow, the environment, and other important aspects of our world. Typically, there are three underlying feelings behind someone's controlling tendencies, which are: fear, unworthiness, and distrust. With fear, we worry that things will not turn out as we want or that something bad will happen. For example, you call your son daily to make sure he's doing okay even though he's requested less contact. With unworthiness, which is connected to shame, we convince ourselves that we do not deserve support and that things will not go our way and, instead, we deserve to suffer and control serves to decrease apparent suffering, while in reality it may be increasing it. For example, in a relationship that is dysfunctional with lots of conflict, the people convince themselves it is better to stay and keep their partner happy in any way that they can. This only serves to aggravate the relationship issues as well as the individual resentment, sadness, pain, and shame. With distrust, we may be scared to let go and count on others, as it may not have worked out well in the past. We begin to believe that we have to manage every aspect of the situation, relationship, or conversation; otherwise, it will not go the way we want. For example, not asking for help with the housework, as you don't trust anyone to do it the way you want.

Write about how the feelings of fear, unworthiness and distrust apply in situations where you want to have control.

_____

_____

_____

_____

_____

In reality, all of us need to rely on faith, our own self-worth and trust in others to move forward in life. Trust requires honesty, which may be difficult if addictive thinking scripts are running in the mind in a distorted manner, minimizing certain aspects and catastrophizing other aspects.

It can be difficult to identify addictive thinking within the self, but easier to spot in others. However, hearing and seeing it in others generates feelings and reactions, as well as information.

How do you feel when you hear addictive thinking in others?

_____

_____

_____

_____

_____

Common responses are:

- Feeling confused/puzzled
- Feeling irritated/annoyed/angry
- Amused, able to laugh about it
- Feeling physically upset (e.g., sick in the stomach)

Addictive thinking is the conglomeration of irrational, distorted thoughts that are part of the disease. It perpetuates exaggerated or irrational thought patterns that prolong the effects of psychological states, especially depression and anxiety. It can generate feelings of chaos, anxiety, anger, frustration, upset, discomfort, and feel like you are on the hamster wheel. Addictive thinking starts with an initial thought that quickly snowballs from there. Addictive thinking precedes the behavioural part of Addiction and precipitates all relapse behaviours as mentioned in the previous chapter with cognitive relapse.

ADDICTIVE THINKING AND RECOVERY

Holistic recovery is a framework for developing awareness of addictive thinking and lessening the impact it has on daily living. A goal of treatment with all addictive thinking is to increase awareness of distorted perceptions, talk about the feelings, and take recovery action. Awareness alone is not enough; it is the commitment to recovery action, which in turn creates more awareness and change that are necessary for growth.

What are your disease's key features of addictive thinking?

_____

_____

_____

_____

_____

How do you feel when addictive thinking is active?

_____

_____

_____

_____

_____

TOOLS TO DEAL WITH ADDICTIVE THINKING

The disease of Addiction uses addictive thinking to its advantage as it reinforces feelings of shame and low self-worth by amplifying destructive thinking. It sabotages thinking and feeling and revolves around the predominant belief that

'I am bad.' Talking and getting feedback is valuable to increase self-awareness, as we all have blind spots that we may be unable to see but others can. Here are some additional tools to help you deal with addictive thinking.

Journaling: is a way to process feelings and sometimes gain clarity about disease thinking. Journaling is a powerful tool for helping us work through our thoughts as well. Thinking about something gives us many ideas, but it is often in the writing of those ideas that we can start to see patterns emerge. Through these patterns, we begin to discover who we really are and change the things in our life that are not working. In addition, journaling helps us keep track of our insights, making it a continual process in which we enhance, refine, and expand our ideas and help us identify the things that may be holding us back but also, how to address them in a positive, concrete way. Writing about stressful events helps one come to terms with them, thus reducing the impact of these stressors on overall health. When we bottle up thoughts and feelings for too long, we can become ill due to the adverse effects on the immune system. The field of psychoneuroimmunology is devoted to the study of these connections. To get healthy and stay that way, we generally have to get to the root of our repressed feelings and release them. Writing helps remove mental blocks and allows us to use all of our brainpower to better understand ourselves, others, and the world around us.

Tips for journaling: Journaling will be most effective if it is done daily for at least twenty minutes. Begin anywhere and forget about spelling and punctuation. Privacy is key if you are to write without censor. Write quickly, as this frees your brain from 'shoulds' and other blocks to successful journaling. If it helps, pick a theme for the day, week, or month (for example, peace of mind, confusion, change, shame, or anger). The most important rule of all is that there are no rules.

Take time to practice free-flowing writing for 20 minutes in a journal, notepad or whatever else you choose:

It can be helpful to end a journaling session by focusing on gratitude.

Three things I am grateful for today. (Be specific. For example, that someone opened a door for me today or I heard back from a friend I was waiting for a response from):

1.

2.

3.

Relaxation: There are many techniques for relaxation. Relaxation methods are designed to help a person attain a state of increased calmness and reduce levels of anxiety, stress, or anger. With relaxation, the goal is to achieve a conscious, slow relaxation of all the major muscle groups and activity of the body to stimulate the relaxation response. This includes deeper, slower breathing, decreased muscle tension, lowered blood pressure, and lowered heart rate. Typically, when the body starts to relax, the mind follows suit with diminished anxiety, stress, or anger.

Tips for relaxation: When stressed or anxious, practice deeper, slower, consistent breathing by inhaling for a count of four, holding for a count of two, then exhaling for a count of four (all through the nose, which adds a natural resistance to the breath. You could also breathe in through the nose, out through the mouth). This slow, equal breathing helps calm the nervous system, reduces anxiety and stress, and increases focus by providing more oxygen to the brain.

You can also try progressive muscle relaxation to help reduce muscle tension from head to toe. To start, close your eyes and focus on tensing then relaxing each muscle group for two to three seconds each. Start with the feet and toes, move up to the knees, thighs, glutes, abdominal muscles, stomach, chest, arms, hands, neck, jaw, eyes, and forehead all while maintaining deep, slow breaths.

Try practicing this relaxation strategy now. Notice and write about how you felt before, during and after.

_____

_____

_____

_____

_____

_____

_____

Meditation: can be accompanied by varying degrees of relaxation, but that is not the goal, only a side effect. Meditation is a mental discipline in which the individual creates an intention to move beyond thinking into a deeper, more profound state of awareness and transcendental state. With meditation, one can achieve better self-knowledge, clarity of thought, lowered stress, improved health, greater focus, and overall well-being. There are other practices, which some may call meditation, such as contemplation, which is reflecting on some positive thoughts, and concentration, which involves focusing the mind on specific ideas. It must be appreciated that contemplation and concentration are more focused on control or substitution of thoughts, whereas true meditation is a process of letting go, acceptance, and orienting towards alignment with the functioning of the rest of the universe. Control or substitution can bring temporary relief by shifting focus; however, true relief comes with a discipline that involves acceptance of all that is without judgement or desire to fix. This acceptance also connects with equanimity (mental calmness and evenness), which allows one to not get caught in judgement by labelling things 'good' or 'bad' but able to see the balance in everything.

Tips for meditation: Sit in a comfortable position with your back supported, if needed. Close your eyes and make no effort to control the breath; simply breathe deeply and naturally. To relax your body, you can use progressive muscle relaxation, to relax your mind, allow your thoughts to wander, rather than trying to control or influence them. When you become aware of thoughts or feelings that arise, and they will, let them go rather than stay engaged. Many people find it beneficial to repeat a mantra (a sound or word that has no meaning or association for you, such as 'om') or return the focus back to breath to help return to a state of relaxed awareness. Meditation is most effective when done daily. You can start by meditating for two to five minutes and then gradually increase the time to 20 minutes. Transcendental Meditation® is a specific technique that provides you with a mantra (sound) to help your brain connect with transcendental consciousness and is recommended to be practiced two times per day.

Take time to practice this meditation exercise now or come back to it after completing the next section of the workbook. Process your experience here by writing down challenges, benefits, and how it felt to take this time for meditation.

_____

_____

_____

_____

_____

_____

ADDICTIVE THINKING AND RELAPSE

It has been well documented in our experience that addictive thinking precedes the use of substances or behaviours and precipitates relapse. As discussed in the relapse continuum section from earlier in the book, relapse happens long before people act out with substance use or behaviour. Noticing a flare-up in addictive thinking, as evidenced by any of the features described in this chapter, is a warning sign that Addiction is active and could progress and manifest in other ways. In addition to addictive thinking, it is also important to pay attention to the spiritual, emotional, biological, and behavioural symptoms you are experiencing.

If an individual is unaware of these relapse warning signs, they will continue down the slippery slope and eventually act out or use. Often people are puzzled by what precipitated their relapse but addictive thinking provides information about how active the disease is. It is often difficult to identify addictive thinking in oneself; therefore, the importance of connecting with trusted friends, family, people in healthy recovery, and health care professionals who understand Addiction is essential.

What recovery action are you willing to take to deal with addictive thinking?

_____

_____

_____

_____

_____

_____

_____

THE JOHARI WINDOW

The Johari Window is a helpful tool to increase self-awareness. The concept was created by two psychologists, Mr. Joseph Luft and Mr. Harrington Ingham, to help people better understand their relationships with themselves and others. Luft and Ingham called their construct 'Johari' after combining parts of their first names. The Johari Window is illustrated as a 2x2 grid. It distinguishes what people can or cannot see in themselves and what others can or cannot see in them. It is useful to increase self-awareness, personal development, and interpersonal relationships. The Johari Window (Figure 1) focuses on four basic aspects of the self: The public self (open); the private hidden self (secret); the blind self (blind spots); and the undiscovered self (unknown).

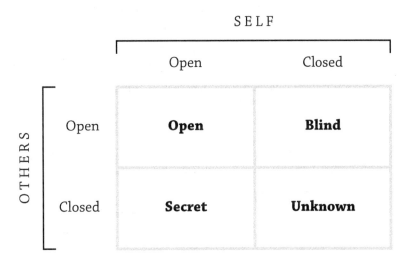

The *public/open self* is what you and others see in you. You typically do not mind discussing this part of yourself with others. Most of the time you agree with this view you have and others have of you. A goal of therapy is to increase the size of the open area by decreasing the blind spots. This is done by being receptive to feedback from others. This is a goal for a healthy, holistic recovery. Life and self becomes transparent, as there is no longer a need for deceit, lying, or manipulation.

Describe some of your characteristics and traits. You can also ask people around you for feedback on what they see as some of your core features.

_____

_____

_____

_____

_____

The *hidden or secret self* is what you see in yourself but others do not. In this part, you hide things that are very private about yourself. You may not want this information to be disclosed for your own protection. It could also be that you may be ashamed of these areas due to vulnerability and to having your perceived faults and dysfunctions exposed. A goal of therapy is to move hidden information, thoughts, and feelings into the open area through the process of disclosure. By telling others how you feel and other information about yourself, you reduce the hidden area and increase the open area, which enables better understanding and trust. With Addiction, the disease is trying to protect itself, which is often shame-driven, and "we are as sick as our secrets."

Write down some obvious secrets that you are keeping. Also write down some things that have happened, recently or in the past that you viewed as insignificant, unimportant and/or shameful. These may be part of your hidden self.

_____

_____

_____

_____

_____

*If you have a sponsor, you may want to consider sharing some of this information with them or someone else you trust as this helps move the information from the hidden to the open pane of the window.

The *blind self* is what is known by others, but is unknown to us. We cannot see what we cannot see. A blind area could include issues that others are deliberately withholding from a person. By seeking or soliciting feedback from others, the aim is to reduce the blind pane and thereby increase the open area to promote self-awareness. Others can see and hear addictive thinking and behaviour and feedback is important, whether the individual is open to it or not.

Are you receptive to feedback from others?

_____

_____

_____

_____

_____

When and by whom?

_____

_____

_____

_____

_____

Do you agree with how they describe you?

_____

_____

_____

_____

_____

The *undiscovered or unknown self* is part of ourselves that you cannot see, nor can others around you, as it is part of our unconscious awareness. Examples of unknown factors may include a natural ability or aptitude that a person does not realize they possess; an unconscious fear or aversion; repressed feelings; or conditioned behaviours or attitudes from childhood. The processes by which this information and knowledge can be uncovered are various and can be prompted through self-discovery, observation by others, or collectively through mutual discovery within a group setting. Psychotherapy helps uncover unknown issues when therapeutically appropriate. As with disclosure and soliciting feedback, the process of self-discovery is a sensitive one. The extent and depth to which an individual is able to seek out and discover their unknown feelings are at the individual's own discretion. Some people are more keen and able than others to do this. The unknown area could also include repressed or subconscious feelings rooted in formative events and traumatic past experiences, which can stay unknown for a lifetime.

How do you feel about self-exploration? Write more about any fear, excitement, hope, shame, sadness, optimism, resentment, and more that you may be experiencing right now.

_____

_____

_____

_____

_____

With Addiction, the individual is being deceived by their brain. Everyone around them is being fooled too. This deception can manifest as lying for no reason, or not even being aware that one is lying. For example, someone saying, "I tried to call to tell you I would be late", though no call was made or believing that they are doing well and coping just fine, though outward evidence would say otherwise. The brain gets so used to living in a constant state of shame and fear it automatically generates stories and excuses as a cover. Information in the unknown pane, with time and recovery, can move into the hidden, blind, or open pane. Staying in the process of recovery will reveal things that may have been hidden for a long time.

Do you do or say things that are not necessarily true and have no idea why? If so, provide some examples.

_____

_____

_____

_____

_____

Have you had vague feelings or memories that you cannot identify clearly? Please write down whatever you remember, especially the feelings, and then talk to someone in your recovery circle or a professional knowledgeable about Addiction.

_____

_____

_____

_____

_____

_____

SELF-TALK

We constantly have dialogue within our minds that informs everything, including how we act and feel about ourselves. This is called self-talk. Self-talk is a helpful tool in recovery and self-development as it is something we can change over time, for with awareness comes action and with action comes change. Here we encourage you to take some time to become acquainted with your inner dialogue and tune in to the conversation.

What do you say to yourself about yourself? Write down specific language and statements and as many as you can identify. For example, "I am such an idiot" or "I am working on getting better at this" or "Dumbass"

_____

_____

_____

_____

_____

What do you say to yourself about Addiction? List as many words and statements as possible.

_____

_____

_____

_____

_____

_____

_____

What do you say to yourself about recovery? List as many words and statements as possible.

_____

_____

_____

_____

_____

_____

_____

_____

What do you say to yourself about others? (e.g., judgments, compliments, envy)

_____

_____

_____

_____

_____

What is the typical focus of your self-talk in a day? (e.g., yourself, criticism, judgments of others, work, hobbies, distraction).

_____

_____

_____

_____

_____

Self-talk can be destructive when steeped in fear and shame; or it can support healthy levels of self-esteem and self-worth when rooted in reality, which serves as the antidote to the powerful feeling of shame that Addiction generates in great quantities. If someone is living in shame, they are likely having thoughts generated through their self-talk that support these feelings. For example, that they are useless, fat, ugly, unworthy, unlovable, or flawed. This is where self-talk, particularly if not honestly attended to, can erode self-worth and perpetuate low self-esteem, shame, anxiety, depression, and potentially many other uncomfortable feelings.

As we grow up, we hear messages, both direct and indirect from parents, siblings, guardians, teachers, peers, and others in our lives. Without even knowing it, we take on some of these messages as our own. When exploring self-talk, people will often be surprised to realize that a message they give to themselves is something that their mother, brother, teacher or other used to say to them.

Can you identify any external sources of the self-talk statements that you listed above?

_____

_____

_____

_____

_____

_____

Do you agree with the self-talk statements you wrote down in the previous questions? Where do you disagree?

_____

_____

_____

_____

_____

_____

_____

Self-talk is something that can be changed and have tremendous benefit. As self-worth increases, feelings of shame, unworthiness, sadness, depression, anxiety, fear, loneliness, and isolation diminish. Over time, self-talk can focus on gratitude, accomplishment, strength, and affirmation.

We can continue to build awareness of our self-talk by doing the exercise below repeatedly. This helps clarify the situations that trigger thoughts and what feelings these thoughts generate. Over time, we can then explore the thoughts or self-talk to see if it is real and fits for us. If not, then we can disengage from it and introduce new dialogue. For example, we can move from thinking "I have nothing to offer in a relationship" to "I have many strengths and traits, including kindness, caring, thoughtfulness, and respect that are beneficial to me and others. I am valuable." The latter thought will come with very different feelings than the former. For now, let us cultivate awareness.

List SITUATIONS that have occurred recently or in the past that you can identify trigger strong thoughts and feelings:

_____

_____

_____

_____

_____

_____

_____

List some of your THOUGHTS related to these situations:

_____

_____

_____

_____

_____

_____
_____

Now write your FEELINGS:

_____
_____
_____
_____
_____
_____
_____

Addiction, being a brain disease, affects feelings, memory, motivation, learning, reward circuitry, spirituality and, of course, thinking. The disease of Addiction uses self-talk to its advantage by reinforcing feelings of shame and low self-worth. It does this by amplifying the 'shoulda, coulda, woulda' talk and focusing on what is wrong or bad about the person, rather than on strengths and what is going well. For example, "I should be further along in my recovery" or "I could have done recovery earlier in life if I was not in that unhealthy job" or "I would be healthier if not for my family of origin."

List your 'shoulda, coulda, wouldas':

"I should ..."

_____
_____
_____
_____
_____

"I could ..."

_____
_____
_____
_____
_____

"I would ..."

_____
_____
_____
_____
_____

With Addiction, it may be impossible to know consistently as to what thoughts are fed by the diseased part of the brain and which are fed by the rational, healthy part of the self. The diseased brain can be very tricky and can make the person in recovery believe the negative statements. This is exactly why it is impossible to do recovery on one's own. Receiving feedback on how much you are living in your thinking is important, as Addiction has a tendency to intellectualize everything and avoid feelings. When exploring self-talk, it is important to look at the feelings that are being generated by your internal dialogue. Feelings are the best guide to telling you if you are on the recovery side of things, so having regular check-ins with yourself about how you feel is a useful daily tool; and checking it in with others who you trust in recovery is also important.

Healthy Self-Talk

- *If you are working on conscious self-talk, than you are practicing recovery talk*

- *Automatic thoughts may be generated by the disease so be careful! Don't buy in to what your disease is selling you*

- *Here is where 'script writing' occurs – anticipating the future, coming up with lots of different scenarios that may or may not happen and feeling them as though they are real.*

Practicing healthy self-talk, or shifting self-talk in a healthy direction, is both simple and complex. The complexity comes from the overwhelming number of thoughts we have in a day, which all come with associated feelings and, at times, behaviours. The simplicity is in the tool: our thoughts are ours alone and only we have access to them. If we listen, get support, and practice, then shifting self-talk is possible.

There are numerous books written about self-talk, implications, and the 'how-to' of making change, but in a nutshell the process is to:

- *Start paying attention and gain more awareness of your thoughts;*

- *Connect with the feelings generated by these thoughts;*

- *Identify the thoughts that are not serving health or recovery;*

- *Develop healthy alternatives to the common self-defeating thoughts, e.g., "I'm so dumb, why didn't I pay more attention" to "I'm doing the best I can, I will pay more attention the next time";*

- *Practice catching and challenging your thinking and implementing the healthy alternatives over time.*

Journaling or writing down the thoughts is the most straightforward way to develop clarity and awareness around your thinking, as you started to practice earlier. It is important to be specific with the language and connect with the exact words that you use to describe yourself or reflect on a situation. This supports the other steps of identifying and shifting self-talk because it gives you concrete examples to work with. The awareness will likely take at least a few weeks to gain a solid footing in as it is important to allow yourself to encounter various situations and challenges to see how your thinking responds. Keep a daily journal or write thoughts down as you notice them. You may begin to see patterns, or certain ways of thinking in response to certain events, or it may seem like a random mixture of thoughts. Either is fine, the important part is to be connected to your inner dialogue rather than coasting on autopilot.

How do you feel about keeping a daily journal? What are the challenges and benefits?

_____

_____

_____

_____

When journaling the situations and thoughts to gain awareness, it is also important to connect with the feelings that are associated with these events and thoughts. For instance, when thinking "I am such an idiot", you may notice that you feel frustrated at the same time. After being turned down for a promotion and thinking "what is wrong with me?" the resultant feelings may be rejection, disappointment, anger, shame, and sadness. There is no right or wrong when it comes to journaling thoughts and feelings; this is our internal perspective. Identifying and validating the feelings, rather than judging, censoring, or avoiding them, help us build esteem and worth as we begin to support the idea that "I am worth it and my feelings are worthy too". Feelings can come in varying degrees and may seem contradictory (e.g., feeling some contentment and frustration at the same time) but all of it is okay.

Write down your beliefs about feelings. For instance, can we hold feelings of happiness and sadness at the same time? Do we have "good and bad" feelings? Are some feelings better than others? Write any other beliefs you may have.

_____

_____

_____

_____

_____

_____

_____

Once there has been an opportunity to journal thoughts and feelings, it is easier to identify where change may be needed in self-talk. For example, you may notice a particular phrase or statement that you say to yourself repeatedly, such as, "Geez, what is wrong with me?" It may not even be the same statement that keeps being repeated, but a similar message, for instance that "I am less than" or "I am not good enough" that comes up in different situations. The emotional impact of this inner dialogue is likely also clearer by this point. Shame, low self-worth, frustration, depression, or anxiety are just a few potential side effects of these thoughts, which in turn can propel behaviours like isolation, increased errors, lack of motivation, or giving up on projects.

Once you have an idea of where change is needed in your inner dialogue, it is important to look at developing alternative statements or phrases that, over time, can come to replace the talk that is currently there. This can be challenging and support from others in recovery and professionals may be necessary to support this change, as a particular way of thinking can be so ingrained that thinking outside of the box may feel impossible, although it is not.

TAKING ACTION: Once you are aware of how you are thinking, you can start to develop alternative statements to introduce into your thinking.

DEVELOPING ALTERNATIVES

- *Have them be realistic (to you)*

- *Encompass compassion, consideration, and respect*

- *Consider: "What would I say to someone else who was thinking this way?"*

Examples of alternatives may include saying "You are doing the best you can" rather than "You are a useless piece of sh*t." Another example may be "I am taking my recovery day by day" rather than "You need to be better at this." Yet another example may be "I am developing my relationship with my Higher Power" rather than "I don't understand this Higher Power stuff."

Altering internal dialogue involves compassion and acceptance. Some people will use affirmations, which are powerful phrases that carry a great deal of personal meaning. Examples can include: "I am worthy," "I am strong," "I am fearless," "My feelings are my feelings and they are okay." Affirmations can be used to replace self-defeating statements and can also be repeated throughout the day to support a shift towards more compassionate inner dialogue, even in the absence of any disruptive chatter.

DEVELOPING AFFIRMATIONS

Example: "I am such a loser."
Alternative:

_____

Example: "What a waste of time."
Alternative:

_____

Example: "No one loves me."
Alternative:

_____

Write down your own common self-talk statements and some healthier alternatives:

Statement:

_____

Alternative:

_____

Statement:

_____

Alternative:

_____

Statement:

_____

Alternative:

_____

Statement:

_____

Alternative:

_____

Statement:

_____

Alternative:

_____

Develop a list of 10 affirmations that you can incorporate into your self-talk and recovery.

1.

2.

3.

4.

5.

6.

7.

8.

9.

10.

*"Daily practice and attention will need to be paid to your thinking for at least
one month until the habit starts to become more natural."*

Once you have decided to explore self-talk, it important to build this into your daily self-care routine and create reminders for yourself to journal, write out situation-thoughts-feelings, and develop and use affirmations. Daily practice and attention will need to be paid to your thinking for at least one month until the habit starts to become more natural. This does not mean the process ends or finishes after one month but, at this time, the tools you have been using to address your self-talk will be more routine and require less overt energy and time. The work, however, will continue as recovery is a process.

Key messages

- Distortion in thinking, also known as addictive thinking, is not unique to Addiction and all of us can be challenged by our own cognitive distortions. This typically occurs when we feel insecure, have low self-esteem, feel stressed, and have difficulty adjusting to life's challenges.

- Addictive thinking does not necessarily indicate Addiction, but greater intensity and regularity of this type of thinking is most common among people with the disease.

- Addictive thinking is irrational, distorted thoughts that can manifest as all-or-nothing thinking, rationalization, denial, minimization, hypersensitivity/reactivity, the illusion of control, morbid expectations, and catastrophizing. Addictive thinking propagates feelings of guilt and shame in the person experiencing them.

- Addictive thinking generally precedes the use of substances or addictive behaviours and precipitates relapse. Holistic recovery is a framework for developing awareness of addictive thinking and lessening the impact it has on daily living.

- A goal in treatment for addictive thinking is to increase awareness of distorted perceptions, talk about the feelings, and take recovery action. Awareness alone is not enough and it is the commitment to recovery action, which in turn creates more awareness and the change necessary to grow.

- Increased self-awareness occurs by talking and getting feedback from those we trust, as we all have blind spots that we may be unable to see or hear—but others can.

- The Johari Window, a technique used in counselling, helps increase self-awareness and allows people to better understand their relationship with themselves and others.

- Self-talk is another valuable tool for health and wellness development, a term used to refer to the ongoing, internal conversation that we have with ourselves and is beneficial to explore as part of recovery from Addiction.

- Developing awareness and practicing healthy self-talk can lead to benefits in many areas, including dealing with stress more effectively, exploring feelings honestly, and improving self-worth and esteem.

Action steps for Chapter 3 (follow through after chapter exercises)

In this chapter, you explored your disease's distorted thinking and self-talk. Moving forward, it will be important to continue your exploration and awareness of your addictive thinking. Every time you become aware of addictive thinking, make a note or journal entry so you can start to see patterns. What are the people, places and things that are triggering your addictive thinking? This awareness will help you become better acquainted with your disease and learn about its symptoms and activators.

Chapter 4: Addictive Feeling

"Many of us spend our whole lives running from feeling with the mistaken belief that you cannot bear the pain.
But you have already borne the pain. What you have not done is feel all you are beyond that pain."
—*Kahlil Gibran*

One of the characteristics of Addiction is the "dysfunctional emotional response" ('E' of the disease). What this really means is that people with Addiction struggle to identify, feel, and express feelings in a proactive, consistent, and healthy way. Addiction creates many internal obstacles to feeling the feelings, including minimization, exaggeration, avoidance, control, fear, and numbness. Developing a connection with your emotional world is a key step to health for anyone and is incredibly important when Addiction is involved. If avoidance of feelings (which is generated by the disease) continues to run the show then ongoing abstinence and recovery becomes difficult, if not impossible. It may take you a long time to feel comfortable with the material in this chapter. That is okay. Be patient, gentle, and open with yourself to keep exploring and delving into the world of feelings and emotions. It may be uncomfortable at times, but it is definitely worth it (just like you are).

"Feelings are just feelings, they are neither good nor bad, they are just information."

FEELINGS AND EMOTIONS

Feelings are the conscious, subjective experience of the core emotions of fear, anger, joy, disgust, and sadness, which have many emotional offshoots including hesitation, paranoia, frustration, rage, apprehension, happiness, contentment, repulsion, depression, melancholy. Feelings are actually felt and experienced (hence the terminology of 'feelings' because you feel it in your senses). Emotions are constantly being generated throughout the day while one is alone or interacting with others. Every interaction, thought, experience, and activity comes with an emotional response, whether we are aware of it at the feelings level or not. Emotions can be conscious or unconscious and 'emoting' is just an expression of the emotions through feelings. Emotions can be alive and well but we may not always be aware of them. Part of the work needed for emotional health, then, is to take time to move emotions from the unconscious to conscious level of awareness. It is hard to heal and sit with feelings if we do not even know what is there!

Initially, it may seem difficult to move emotions from an unconscious level to a conscious, feelings level. The purpose of this chapter in the workbook is to give you some specific awareness questions and action steps to work through to continue increasing your emotional knowledge and expression.

Make a list of feelings that you can identify within yourself, past and present.

_____

_____

_____

_____

_____

_____

_____

This list of feelings would be helpful to keep handy and to use for your daily feelings check-in. You can refer to this list when journaling to connect with how things felt for you that day, rather than just focusing on what happened. Here are some additional feelings words that you can add to your own list if they resonate for you.

Happy	Fear	Joy	Content
Frustration	Irritable	Love	Peace
Greed	Lust	Jealousy	Affection
Loss	Ignorant	Envy	Shame
Grief	Stupid	Satisfied	Vengeful
Anger	Useless	Worried	Claustrophobic
Sadness	Wasteful	Prideful	Trapped
Depressed	Achieved	Empathy	Abnormal
Anxious	Interested	Ecstasy	Unusual
Stress	Eager	Judgemental	Amused
Overwhelmed	Virtuous	Compassion	Abandoned
Confused	Worried	Equanimity	Searching
Tense	Helpless	Relieved	Seeking
Scared	Ambitious	Balanced	Euphoric
Desiring	Cynical	Guilty	Restless
Craving	Threatened	Fulfilled	Bewildered
Empty	Generous	Weak	Centred
Blue	Lonely	Energized	Whole
Cheerful	Satisfied	Giddy	Fragmented
Fatigue	Gentle	Tired	Broken
Surrender	Fragile	Delight	Aware
Hope	Careful	Pleasure	Spiritual
Faith	Distracted	Rejected	Egotistic
Confident	Disappointed	Relief	Small
Cautious	Dissatisfied	Pressure	Inspired
Hesitant	Apathy	Controlled	Alert
Strong	Sorry	Controlling	Astounded
Nurturing	Forgiving	Inauthentic	Awe
Caring	Resentment	Deprived	Foolish
Comfortable	Disgust	Discomfort	Glad
Stuffed	Playful	High	Glee

Authentic	Lost	Connected	Bored
Disenchanted	Frazzled	Manipulated	Tired
Kind	Aroused	Flat	Childish
Grace	Terrified	Deceived	Valued
Placid	Rage	Betrayed	Ambivalent
Calm	Numb	Forced	Engaged
Attentive	Nervous	Coerced	Betrayed
Aware	Silly	Victim	Pity
Aggressive	Hostile	Regret	Adamant
Bitchy	Competitive	Hopeless	Lazy
Destructive	Isolated	Pain	Panicked
Deceitful	Precarious	Shy	Solemn

How do you see using this list of feelings to support your recovery?

_____

_____

_____

_____

_____

What challenges and barriers are coming up for you as you start to explore the topic of feelings? What information do these reactions provide?

_____

_____

_____

_____

_____

_____

_____

CORE EMOTIONS WITH ADDICTION

Shame. This is the experience of feeling fundamentally flawed, useless, or unworthy. It is a profoundly deep and overarching feeling that is more widespread than a feeling such as guilt, which is usually tied to a specific event that we feel bad about. For example, a person might feel guilty for yelling at their child when they were tired. For someone carrying shame, they would take this event as more evidence of their inability to be a parent and of how awful they are as a human being. Everyone has shame, but some people have it more than others. For those who have Addiction, it is critical to explore feelings of shame as this is a major generator of disease activity. In order for people to stabilize in recovery, processing and healing from their shame is a core part of the process. Doing this involves putting those parts of you that you carry shame about into the light, which means to out them to others, as well as yourself.

Make a list of all the 'deep, dark' secrets that you have been carrying throughout your life. This is a list of what you believe are the worst things that you have ever thought, said, or done to self or others. Write them down even if you have shared these secrets with others (there can never be too much light shed on our shame):

_____

_____

_____

_____

_____

_____

_____

Reflect on how you would feel sharing these secrets with another person. What would you fear? What would you look forward to?

_____

_____

_____

_____

_____

_____

_____

Who would be the safest person to share these secrets with? (In other words, who would be most likely to be compassionate, empathetic, and non-judgemental? This can be a friend, family member, fellow person in recovery, sponsor, counsellor, or spiritual mentor).

_____

_____

_____

_____

_____

_____

What makes this person the safest for you?

_____

_____

_____

_____

Would you be willing to challenge yourself to share some of the information on your list above with this safe person? How come and, if not, what are the barriers?

_____

_____

_____
_____
_____

It is only through outing those parts of ourselves that we carry the most shame about that we have the opportunity to heal. If we try and build self-esteem in other ways, such as by using affirmations, emotional awareness, spiritual counsel, and reinforcing self-talk, but still hang on to secrets that we believe mark us as flawed and terrible, then these other tools will not be of maximum benefit. This is something that takes time and having safe people around to share with. If you do not have a safe person at this point in time, that is okay, but please keep in mind the importance of getting open and honest in the future to keep developing your recovery. As the saying goes, "We are only as sick as our secrets".

When you are ready to challenge yourself to be more open about your shame, it is essential to have an emotional self-care plan in place. Identify what would be most calming and relaxing for you before and after having such a conversation (e.g., going to a 12-Step meeting, journaling, meditating, taking a bubble bath, going for a walk, reading, being with others or being alone to process).

Before:

_____
_____
_____
_____
_____

After:

_____
_____
_____
_____
_____

Shame is the deepest and most toxic emotion that drives addictive thinking and behaviour. This makes it one of the most uncomfortable feelings to process through, but also one of the most relieving and rewarding as this work gets done. In recovery, people come to recognize that they will always have some shame in them, but it is profoundly freeing to have this lessen over time. We encourage you to open up to safe people, in the context of a self-care plan, as you feel ready to do so. Taking the step to be more open with yourself is a big one in and of itself.

Fear. As with the other emotions, fear is designed to provide us with information. Fear tells us when we are coming up against a challenge that is unfamiliar and uncertain to us and we have no way of predicting the outcome. Our brains may tell us we need to figure out the outcome before we move through whatever we are afraid of, which is of course impossible, but this can keep people stuck in inaction for a long time. It is important to gain awareness of where we are carrying fear and work on taking action through it.

What are the biggest challenges you are facing at this time?

_____

_____

_____

_____

_____

List the fears that come up in facing these challenges:

_____

_____

_____

_____

_____

What other feelings are coming up in addition to fear?

_____

_____

_____

_____

_____

When we are dealing with fear, it is important to develop an honest and realistic appreciation of what is important to us. We can stay where we are for a long time, but usually we reach a point where the pain of changing becomes less than the pain of staying the same.

What would be most important to you if today was your last day on earth? Who you would you want to be with? What would you want to do? What would you say to those around you? What fears would be less important?

_____

_____

_____

_____

_____

_____

_____

Where can you challenge yourself to change? List one thing that you can do differently to live in accordance with who you are and what you believe (which are your answers to the last question). Be specific about what this will look like and when it will happen or start.

_____

_____

_____

_____

_____

Control related to fear and shame. When we are experiencing the uncomfortable emotions of fear and shame, the disease of Addiction is happy to try and take over with various 'solutions' to make these feelings go away. Control is one of these strategies. Control is the illusion that we have the ability to influence something. If we can control the person, situation, or feeling itself then we are okay, right? Unfortunately this does nothing to address the feelings or situations generating them. It is important to recognize what, when, and how we are trying to use control to avoid our feelings so that we can move towards feeling those feelings instead. Control is about *making* something happen, rather than allowing it to happen as it needs to.

Circle the examples below that illustrate control:

Avoiding something

Booking appointments for someone

Giving the silent treatment

Excessive talking

Keeping very busy

Micromanaging

Criticism/judgement

Keeping a 'scorecard' in relationships

Withholding love or affection

Unwilling to listen to others

Not sharing my true feelings

Telling someone how to act

Using passive-aggression

Black and white thinking

Lying

Asking many, many questions

Isolation

Conditional acceptance/caring

Snooping, spying

Jealousy

Belittling, arguing, name-calling

Going along with other's plans

All of these are examples of control. Control does not just involve directly trying to modify or alter another person or a situation (like telling someone what to do or how they need to change, or being critical of them). Control can be just as powerful in our avoidance or lack of action. For instance, when we are giving someone the silent treatment or not sharing our true feelings then we may be trying to avoid conflict and 'not rock the boat'. We are assuming that by not saying anything, the outcome will be that everyone is happy, which is obviously not the case because you are not happy, for one, and the other(s) may not be either. Control can be very subtle. Many people may not think they are controlling when, in fact, their disease may often take them there. Here are some additional questions to get you exploring your relationship with control.

When you have conversations with others, what expectations do you have for what will happen in the conversation or as a result of the conversation? Write down some specific examples.

Expectations:

Examples:

1.

2.

3.

4.

5.

If these outcomes or expectations do not happen, what do you do?

_____
_____
_____
_____
_____

How do you feel when you do not *have control over a situation, person, or outcome?*

_____
_____
_____
_____
_____

Can you use the Serenity Prayer to reflect on a situation in terms of where you do have some power and where you are powerless? Practice using a pertinent example.

Example:

_____
_____
_____
_____
_____

List the things I cannot change about the person and situation (serenity):

_____
_____
_____
_____
_____

List the things I can change within myself and the situation (courage):

_____
_____
_____
_____
_____

Who can I check this out with to get some additional feedback and support (wisdom)?

_____
_____
_____
_____
_____

Write about your fear of letting go and trusting that things will work out:

_____
_____
_____
_____
_____

Write about the 'coincidences' you have experienced recently or long ago.

_____
_____
_____
_____
_____

Often it is in these 'coincidences' that our Higher Power (HP) is at play. Through developing a stronger relationship with our HP we are then able to let go of control and trust that everything will work out as it needs to, not necessarily as we want it to or as our brains are telling us it should.

As we struggle with control, fear, and shame that we are not paying attention to, they may build up and result in anger.

Anger. Anger is a core emotion and needs to be treated as such, rather than referred to as a 'secondary' emotion where it sometimes get misinterpreted as being less important than others. It is true that anger is often connected to other feelings, but we can (and need to) feel anger in and of itself. Anger informs us when we have been violated in some way; when our needs are not being met or an internal boundary has been crossed. For example, we become angry when we are continuously being treated disrespectfully – our internal boundary of how we know we deserve to be treated has been violated.

Make a list (and continue to add to it over time) of your internal boundaries, morals, values, ethics, and beliefs about behaviour (e.g., not swearing in conversation, never hitting people, being treated with respect and compassion):

_____
_____
_____
_____
_____
_____
_____

When was the last time you can recall feeling angry? Describe the situation, how your body felt, what you were thinking at the time, other feelings you could connect with, and how you dealt with that feeling of anger.

_____
_____
_____
_____
_____
_____
_____

What internal boundaries were being violated in this situation to propel anger?

_____
_____
_____
_____
_____

It is important to move towards assertive language in dealing with boundary violations that can generate anger. Assertiveness means using "I" language in expressing feelings and thoughts, rather than "you" language. For example, "I am feeling hurt" rather than "Why did you hurt me?" When we are being assertive we are clearly stating our feelings without being attached to an outcome. We are sharing for the purpose of expression, not to change behaviour or the situation. In terms of communication, anger can also propel us into passiveness (not saying anything at all) or aggression (saying how we feel in an attacking, judging, or vengeful way). We can also become passive-aggressive, which is the dance between keeping the feelings in and having them explode in a way that is counterproductive.

How could you use assertiveness to handle the situation you wrote about before that generated anger? Remember that assertiveness involves using "I" language, not focusing on the behaviour or blame, and incorporating feelings. Write down what you could say using "I feel _____ when" _____.

_____

_____

_____

_____

_____

It is not uncommon when people try to practice being assertive to say " I felt angry when YOU_____, this is still attaching blame to another rather than expressing how you feel. A healthier interaction is "I feel angry when I'm ignored."

You are doing great work looking honestly at your feelings of shame, fear, and anger. Doing this work is incredibly rewarding and valuable and, as you do it, you will be able to connect with additional emotions, including that of joy.

Joy. This is the feeling of great pleasure or happiness that comes when we are doing something enjoyable that matches our authentic self. The word 'enjoyable' identifies people, places and things that one can get joy from through connection. While this emotion is not very predominant (or sometimes even present) in active Addiction, it becomes more bountiful in recovery. To help you connect with your inner joy, here are some activities to try.

Go and sit outside or near a window and spend 10 minutes just observing. Connect with the sights, sounds, smells, and feel of the environment around you. Enjoy just sitting and being.

This activity may be uncomfortable and/or difficult the first few (hundred!) times you try it but connecting with the world around you, particularly nature, and being still creates space for your inner joy to reveal itself. Keeping up a busy pace and lifestyle may feel joyful and rewarding, but it stifles the opportunity for true serenity, which is connected to pure bliss or joy, to come forward. The key to healthy recovery is finding balance between doing and being.

Smile. Research shows that physically raising the corners of our mouths raises our mood. It might feel forced and silly, so try it in private at first if it does, but over time it will come more naturally.

Make a list of healthy, fun activities for you. Build on this list over time as you continue to get to know yourself. (Examples: reading, board games, sporting activities, outdoor activities, arts and crafts.)

_____

_____

_____

_____

_____

Working on awareness and action with the core emotions can help us keep connecting to our inner world of feelings, which offers a wealth of information to us. Below, we continue our exploration of other feelings that you can keep working with.

Feelings to Be Aware Of …

Guilt. This feeling is different from the emotion of shame. Shame is "I am bad" whereas guilt is "I did bad." Guilt is easier to heal from as we can appreciate that the action or event we feel guilty about is not a direct representation of self. For example, if I am upset and lash out, telling someone to leave me alone, I can appreciate that I am human, make mistakes, and was having a vulnerable moment, rather than feeling like that incident represents my awfulness as a human being. In recovery, over time what feels like shame can slowly be shifted to guilt, so away from "I am bad" to "I did bad" and then to acceptance, "I am a fallible human being with many strengths."

Make a list of things you have done that you regret.

_____
_____
_____
_____
_____

Write about how you believe these events make you a bad person:

_____
_____
_____
_____
_____

Of course, these events do not make you a bad person, but shame that has not yet been translated into guilt says they do. In fact, shame says that these events make you a horribly flawed, useless, worthless person, which is counterproductive for health and recovery. With these events that you carry guilt (and likely shame) about, it is important to start to move towards accepting your part in these situations while also being able to see that it was not entirely your fault and to accept that it happened, that you cannot change the past, and that you can 'forgive' yourself for what has happened. This really means accept the things that you cannot change.

Turning these events over to a Higher Power is one way to embrace acceptance. You cannot regret the past, ignore it, or remove it, so one needs to turn to recognition that it happened and appreciation for the gifts it has given you. It is out of your control, it was then and is now, which is the core of turning something over. You let it go and relinquished your perceived sense of power over it, and accepted what was, what is, and what will be.

Develop or write down a prayer that focuses on acceptance. It can be the Serenity Prayer ('God, grant me the serenity to accept the things I cannot change; the courage to change the things I can; and the wisdom to know the difference') or something else you have heard or created.

_____
_____
_____
_____
_____

_____

_____

Say this prayer daily upon rising and just before going to sleep as part of your ongoing routine. Practice it quietly or out loud now for a few minutes.

Resentment. If we do not acknowledge, feel through, and process our anger then it is likely to become solidified as resentment over time. Resentment is our indignant displeasure at having been treated as (what we perceive to be) unfairly.

Make a list of everyone, past and present, that you are carrying resentment towards (e.g., family members, coworkers, childhood friends, teachers, former romantic partners or crushes, self, members of a religious organization or club, anonymous drivers, neighbours, world leaders, fictional characters).

_____

_____

_____

_____

_____

_____

_____

How has this resentment served you? Hurt you?

_____

_____

_____

_____

_____

When we are carrying resentment, it is easier to focus on the other and their inappropriate behaviour than it is to look at our role in a situation. Often, when we are carrying resentment, we have been living with a high degree of expectation. This means that we are looking for specific outcomes with regards to behaviour, situations, and/or the relationship as a whole. For instance, I may expect that someone will stop calling me after 9:00 p.m. if I request that they stop calling me after 9:00 p.m. If they call again at 10:30 p.m. and I feel resentful, that tells me that I was _expecting_ them to listen, rather than viewing it as a request. I have asked them not to call me after 9:00 p.m. but I cannot control their behaviour or thought process. Therefore, it is my responsibility to turn off my phone, put it on silent, or not answer the phone to support my boundary, rather than expecting them to follow through on my boundary.

Make a list of the expectations you can identify having of other people:

_____

_____

_____

_____

_____

_____

_____

Write down each person's name from your resentment list again. Beside their name, write down the expectation(s) you were carrying of them that did not get met:

_____

_____

_____

_____

_____

_____

_____

Now look at each situation and reflect on how you contributed to it. What was your role in generating the outcome you wrote about?

_____

_____

_____

_____

_____

_____

_____

It is important to be appreciative that any relationship is a combination of two people, including their perspectives, feelings, healthy selves, and dysfunctional parts. We can only take responsibility and accountability for our part and must leave the rest to them. We must also look inward at our own expectations of ourselves.

Make a list of the expectations you can identify having of yourself:

_____

_____

_____

_____

_____

Who do you expect yourself to be?

_____

_____

_____

_____

_____

How do you expect yourself to act?

_____

_____

_____

_____
_____

What do you expect your life to look like?

_____
_____
_____
_____
_____

What are the things you expect to avoid being, saying, doing, and having?

_____
_____
_____
_____
_____

How do you feel when your expectations are not met? How do you respond and react?

_____
_____
_____
_____
_____

Looking at your resentment list above, how many of those situations were generated or influenced by your expectations?

_____
_____
_____
_____
_____

Make a list of your boundaries in these situations (e.g., 'Not being name called' or 'not being around substances').

_____
_____
_____
_____
_____
_____

Now make a list of how you can reinforce these boundaries through words and/or action.

_____
_____
_____
_____
_____

_____

_____

It would be our recommendation to share this list of boundaries and reinforcing action with other people in recovery and/or your healthcare providers who are familiar with Addiction as there may be blind spots within your work here that are impossible to see. It is very common that what people believe is a boundary is really an expectation. For example, that people will treat you more respectfully (expectation) rather than taking action to remove yourself from situations where people are being disrespectful (boundary). Also, it is important to discuss with your supports whether reinforcing your boundaries using words is even necessary or if the follow- through really needs to be with action only.

In setting boundaries, we can lose parts of relationships, or even whole relationships, which once felt important to us. This can come with feelings of sadness and loss.

What relationships are you fearful will be impacted if you set boundaries?

_____
_____
_____
_____
_____

How do you fear these relationships will change?

_____
_____
_____
_____
_____

Can you move towards trusting that even if these relationships change or are lost as a result of boundaries, that this indicates this was not a healthy relationship to begin with?

Identifying resentments and your part in them helps slowly bring you closer to acceptance and letting go, which is key for healing from resentment.

What does acceptance look and feel like for you?

_____
_____
_____
_____

Identify the last time you felt accepting of your life and where you were at. Write down the details of this – what was happening, how you felt, how life looked.

_____

_____

_____

_____

_____

_____

_____

What are your fears in letting go of resentment?

_____

_____

_____

_____

_____

How can you practice acceptance and letting go in your life?

_____

_____

_____

_____

_____

_____

_____

As we accept and let go, other feelings may be released, including that of loss, which is common at any point of change or transition. It is important to let the feelings come before you let them go. Trying to accept everything without having a clear appreciation of your feelings is connected to control by avoidance.

Loss. We experience many losses in our lives, not just when people die. Any time something changes, big or little, we experience a sense of loss and transition from what was to what is. Some of these changes are more hurtful and obvious than others, but it is important to feel the feelings with all of them.

Identify the names of people that are no longer in your life that you once had a relationship with.

_____

_____

_____

_____

After writing down these names, take 5 minutes to sit quietly, pen down and eyes closed. Sit with whatever feelings are coming up for you.

Now, having sat with these feelings and sensations, write down how you feel as you reflect on these previous relationships.

_____

_____

_____

_____

_____

What is one healthy thing you can do for self-care right now to show compassion for the loss and other feelings you are experiencing? Take time to do this for yourself.

_____

_____

_____

_____

_____

You have to let all feelings come before you can let them go. Feelings of resentment, loss, and other difficult feelings, including pain, are some of the most difficult to sit with but also the most freeing to let go of. Grief is the feeling we experience when we have lost something or someone that was important. We experience a multitude of losses throughout our lives, even if we have not lost people due to death. Change brings with it a sense of loss. We may not always connect to those feelings of sadness and loss, but they are there. As we grow and change throughout our lives, there are multiple associated losses.

Make a list of the major changes you have experienced in life (moves, new schools, new jobs, children, deaths, recovery dates):

_____

_____

_____

_____

_____

_____

_____

After you have completed this list, take a moment to stop and sit with the feelings that are present. Write the feelings down, then close your eyes and take five minutes to sit quietly. Feel the feelings.

_____

_____

_____

_____
_____
_____

"You have to let all feelings come before you can let them go"

Pain. By definition, all pain is experiential and has an emotional component. As much as there are pain pathways in the peripheral and central nervous system, in chronic pain it is the central nervous system pathways that become significant. There is a direct link between Addiction and perceived physical pain, as the reward circuitry impacted by Addiction is associated with the pain pathways in the brain. Specifically, the brain regions of anterior cingulate gyrus (ACG) and pre-frontal cortex (PFC) are involved in pain perception and emotions.

List the emotions and feelings that are dominant in your awareness when you have physical pain:

_____
_____
_____
_____
_____

Fear? Write about it.

_____
_____
_____
_____
_____

Anger? Write about it.

_____
_____
_____
_____
_____

Shame? Write about it.

_____
_____
_____
_____

It is common to experience despair, frustration, and anxiety that things will get worse rather than better when one is experiencing chronic pain. With addiction-related circuitry being affected, catastrophizing is often present, meaning focusing on worst case scenarios rather than realistic outcomes. Dealing with feelings, especially shame, resentments and worries, helps in living with chronic pain. If you do not have chronic pain, the questions below are relevant even in the context of recovery from Addiction, which generates a lot of pain (emotional and physical).

List the emotions and feelings that are in your awareness when you are experiencing some relief from pain?

_____
_____
_____
_____
_____

How much faith and trust do you have at this time? Write about this.

_____
_____
_____
_____
_____

How much present-moment awareness and acceptance do you have at this time? Write about this.

_____
_____
_____
_____
_____

How much serenity do you have at this time? Write about this.

_____
_____
_____
_____
_____

Pride and Grandiosity. These emotions are used as cover-ups when we are experiencing high levels of shame. Shame tells us that we are bad, so pride and grandiosity are helpful in masking this by focusing on how wonderful our life is, the things we have, and what we have accomplished. Realistically, however, the person carrying high levels of shame does not really believe that these items or accomplishments make them great people, but this is the image that they portray to the world. Over time, if the brain is convincing and the lie great enough, the person with shame may actually believe they have high self-esteem and think well of themselves, but they still have a deep well of shame they are carrying and have not dealt with. Sometimes the blind pane with pride and grandiosity can be so large that it may be difficult for the person living with it to know it exists. Here are some things to reflect on to give you some awareness of where your relationship with yourself is truly at.

Check any of the following statements that apply to you right now.

☐ *I enjoy keeping busy with little down time*

☐ *I find comfort in purchasing material goods, like clothes or other objects*

☐ *I get angry or upset when people give me criticism or constructive feedback*

☐ *I use drugs, alcohol, food, work, exercise, sex, or other behaviours to distract and/or reward and entertain me*

☐ *I use words like 'never' or 'always' to describe my beliefs, morals and life (e.g., "I would never hit someone" or "I always show respect to elders")*

☐ *The people in my life need to change what they are doing*

☐ *I am doing well in my life and do not have much to explore or develop within myself*

☐ *I find myself arguing or getting defensive with others with different opinions than me*

☐ *I strongly dislike and avoid conflict*

☐ *I want my parents or significant others to be proud of me and my accomplishments*

If you checked any of these items, there is a strong likelihood that you are living with shame, avoidance, and denial and are at risk of compensating for this using grandiosity as a cover-up. Endorsing any of these items indicates that there are issues under the surface that you have not explored and that your brain may be preventing you from exploring, which may include feelings or experiences you have not dealt with, or even untreated Addiction or mental health issues. The statements above are representative of the avoidance, escape, and denial strategies that our brains may develop to keep us unwell. Shame can be a difficult emotion to identify and sit with, but once you have outed it, then you can work on being real and letting go of the pride and grandiosity that keep the shame hidden. Once these uncomfortable feelings come out into the light, you can then work on finding different ways of dealing with them.

HEALTHY WAYS OF DEALING WITH FEELINGS

Addiction's primary mode of coping with feelings is using distraction and escape to avoid them. Moving forward in recovery involves sitting with these feelings and facing them, which can be difficult and uncomfortable, as well as unfamiliar. In this section we explore some reflective exercises and activities to get you going on taking the next step into 'feeling the feelings'.

In the past, how have you avoided your feelings? List all activities and behaviours that you can remember from early childhood to present that served to distract you and minimize your feelings (e.g., reading, avoiding conflict, not saying what is on your mind, playing sports, watching TV, video games, accomplishing, distraction through_____.)

_____

_____

_____

_____

_____

What consequences have these activities and behaviours had (on relationships, self, school/work functioning, spiritual health, physical health, thinking, substance use, unhealthy behaviours)?

_____

_____

_____

_____

_____

_____

_____

_____

What are the most uncomfortable feelings for you? List your top five.

1.

2.

3.

4.

5.

What are some behaviours or activities you have tried or could try to help you cope with these and other feelings in a healthy way?

_____

_____

_____

_____

_____

How would these activities or behaviours help? What possible risks or consequences could they have?

_____

_____

_____

_____

_____

What are your hopes and goals in learning to deal with feelings differently?

_____

_____

_____

_____

_____

If you can identify that your hopes are still being motivated by a desire to avoid or escape, then it is important to challenge yourself to sit daily in reflection and experience of your feelings. Here are some activities to push yourself out of the avoidance comfort zone.

Today and for the next week, list all of the feelings that came up for you that day. Focus on 'how' you felt today, not 'what happened'.

Example: Happy, content, frustrated, sad, shame, annoyed, joyful, jealous, sick, depressed, anxious, worried, afraid.

Day 1:

Day 2:

Day 3:

Day 4:

Day 5:

Day 6:

Day 7:

After one week of checking in on feelings, reflect on the challenges as well as benefits of doing this.

One week later – Challenges:

_____

_____

_____

_____

_____

One week later – Benefits:

_____

_____

_____

_____

_____

Can you continue to engage in this daily practice for the next three weeks? This would put you at a whole month of practicing 'feeling the feelings'! If so, come back to reflect on:

One month later – Challenges:

_____

_____

_____

_____

_____

One month later – Benefits:

_____

_____

_____

_____

_____

One month later – Are you likely to keep this activity up?
Yes_____ No_____

One month later – In what ways is your addictive thinking trying to stop you from feeling the feelings?

_____

_____

_____

_____

_____

Key messages

- The content of this chapter contains the foundations for a revolution in your life, health, and recovery. It may take you a long time to work through everything in this chapter and keep expanding upon it, and it will likely bring up lots of uncomfortable feelings along the way but the benefits are profound.

- One of the main goals of recovery is to learn to deal with "life on life's terms", which means dealing with reality as it comes.

- Feelings are our greatest source of information about what is happening in our reality so the more comfortable you can get connecting to them, the more connected you will be to yourself. Take your time with all of the activities in this chapter and beyond, there is no rush to health and well-being, it will come when and as it needs to. If you are finding this work difficult, then slow down and make sure you take time to intersperse fun activities too to provide some levity.

- Recovery is about the journey more than the destination.

Action steps for Chapter 4 (follow through after chapter exercises)

Learning to identify, sit with, process, and communicate feelings is an ongoing and valuable part of the recovery journey. Moving forward, we would encourage you to continue checking in on how you are feeling on a daily basis and using tools like journaling and talking to others to process these. You may want to revisit the material in this chapter and keep reworking it every six months as the feelings and awareness of them will change over time.

Chapter 5: Addictive Behaviour

"We change our behaviour when the pain of staying
the same becomes greater than the pain of changing."
—Henry Cloud

All substances that we ingest affect the body and brain. They may affect us in different ways but, nevertheless, they have an impact. All behaviours that we engage in affect the body and brain. They may affect us in different ways but, nevertheless, they have an impact. Are you noticing a trend? The basic message is that everything we do has an impact on our resultant health and well-being. This chapter is designed to help you start exploring all aspects of substances and behaviours, not just the ones that are obviously problematic and troubling to you, to help give you awareness about where other changes may need to be made to support your ongoing recovery.

ALCOHOL, DRUGS AND BEHAVIOURS IN ADDICTION AND RECOVERY AND THE ROLE OF PRESCRIPTION MEDICATIONS

It is important that you have an overall awareness of all the substances you are putting into your body. Below are lists of substances grouped into their mode of activation (e.g., whether they are stimulants, depressants, and so on). Place a check mark beside all of the substances that you currently use, even if that use is 'recreational' or not daily. If you are currently abstaining from certain substances, it would be worthwhile making note of the substances you are still using and/or the substances that you have used in the past.

Stimulants

☐ Coffee

☐ Caffeinated soft drinks

☐ Tobacco cigarettes

☐ E-cigarette

☐ Methamphetamine (meth or speed)

☐ Crack cocaine

☐ Ritalin (methylphenidate)

☐ Concerta

☐ Vyvanse

☐ Caffeinated tea (green, black, oolong)

☐ Chocolate

☐ Chewing tobacco

☐ Nicotine patches, gum

☐ Crystal meth

☐ MDMA (ecstasy)

☐ Adderall

☐ Cocaine

☐ Energy drinks

Depressants

☐ Alcohol

☐ Clonazepam (Rivotril or Klonopin)

☐ Lorazepam (Ativan)

☐ Zopiclone (Imovane)

☐ Lunesta (eszopiclone)

☐ Any drugs starting with 'Z'

☐ Barbiturates (Luminal, Tuinal, Seconal, Fiorinal)

☐ Propofol

☐ Diazepam (Valium)

☐ Alprazolam (Xanax)

☐ Any drug(s) ending with 'pam'

☐ Ambien (zolpidem)

☐ Sonata, Starnoc (zaleplone)

☐ Seconal

☐ Fiorinal

Opioids

☐ Codeine

☐ Oxycodone

☐ Meperidine (Demerol)

☐ Heroin

☐ Percocet

☐ T1s, T2s, T3s or T4s

☐ Morphine

☐ Hydromorphone (Dilaudid)

☐ Tramadol

☐ Fentanyl

☐ Tramacet

☐ 222s, 282s, 292s

Hallucinogens

☐ Marijuana

☐ Cannabis products

☐ Magic mushrooms

☐ Hash, hash products

☐ LSD

☐ Ketamine

Organic solvents

☐ Glue

☐ Aerosol products

☐ Paint

☐ Paint thinner

☐ Gasoline

Now that you have marked the substances you are currently using, review all of the items you checked and write them down here:

_____

_____

_____

_____

_____

How do you feel seeing these items altogether?

_____

_____

_____

_____

_____

Look at the trends. Are there more checks than you would have anticipated? Are you more vulnerable in one category than another? Write your reflections down.

_____

_____

_____

_____

_____

This activity was designed to give you a heightened level of awareness of the types of substances your brain may desire, as well as see the full array of substances you may be using to mood and mind alter. It is also important to look at other substances and behaviours that your Addiction may be using to seek escape, reward, or relief. Look at the list below and check any behaviours that you are currently engaging in, or have been vulnerable to in the past.

Mood-altering Behaviours

- ☐ Eating until sick
- ☐ VLTs
- ☐ Exercise > 2 hours/day
- ☐ Excessive spending
- ☐ Eating fatty food

- ☐ Using escorts/prostitutes

- ☐ Playing video/cell phone games >2 hours/day

- ☐ Daydreaming regularly

- ☐ Vomiting up food for relief
- ☐ Buying lotto tickets
- ☐ Excessive exercise
- ☐ Working 50+ hours/week
- ☐ Using supplements or over-the-counter products for quick relief

- ☐ Using hook-up apps for sex or fantasy

- ☐ Watching TV >5 hours/day

- ☐ Fantasizing

- ☐ Placing bets on activities
- ☐ Casino gambling
- ☐ Eating sugary treats
- ☐ Eating salty food
- ☐ Pornography and masturbation

- ☐ Cell phone use >1 hour/day

- ☐ Reading > 3 hours/day

- ☐ Thoughts of suicide/escape

The behaviours on this chart, while certainly not exhaustive, gives you an idea of some of the ways your disease may be driving you to find escape, reward, or relief that are not as obvious. We encourage you to be mindful of all behaviours you are engaging in and check them in with people in your support network to get some feedback, both from peers and health-care providers, on whether they are supportive of your recovery. Sometimes abstaining from one aspect of Addiction, for example alcohol, can trigger substitution with food; whereas getting help for obesity in the form of bariatric surgery, especially when Addiction involving food is unrecognized and untreated, can make Addiction involving alcohol more manifest.

What, if any, of the checked substances or behaviours that you are currently engaging in are you willing to move towards abstinence from?

_____

_____

_____

_____

_____

For the substances you wish to be abstinent from, what fears and barriers come up in pursuing abstinence?

_____

_____

_____

_____

_____

If abstinence from that behaviour is not possible (like with food, work, sex, or exercise), it is important to look at the parts of that behaviour that support your recovery and the parts that do not.

What aspects of the behaviour support your recovery? (For example, going into coffee shops or restaurants where sweet treats are not on display if you are vulnerable to acting out with sugar):

_____

_____

_____

_____

_____

What aspects of the behaviour do not *support recovery? (For example, going into bakeries or coffee shops with lots of pastries on display; being alone at supermarket checkouts).*

_____

_____

_____

_____

_____

STAGES OF CHANGE

Behaviour change happens in stages. One needs to consider whether one is in pre-contemplation (there is no problem), contemplation (there is a problem but the person does not know what to do about it), preparation (there is a problem and the person is open to learning what to do), action (there is a problem and the person is doing something about it), or maintenance (significant change has already occurred and now the person is focused on consistency and diligence in routine). It is helpful to look at the barriers to change when one is in the contemplation or preparation stages, using this simple, but profound, 2 x 2 table.

	Benefits	Challenges
Staying the Same		
Changing		

Completing this chart for each substance or behaviour you are looking to change can be enlightening. Below are some examples of the common barriers that people identify.

	Benefits	Challenges
Staying the Same	Box 1: Hits, highs, escape from reality, avoidance, distraction, "fun" (that is really just intoxication)	Box 2: Consequences that are happening (e.g., loss of job, relationship, financial security), detriments to physical and emotional health
Changing	Box 3: Growth opportunities – authenticity, peace, serenity, openness, honesty, joy, happiness, improved health	Box 4: Fear, shame, avoidance, the unknown, resistance from social circle, lack of awareness

Being honest about these barriers allows you to deal with the reality of where Addiction has taken you so far and where it will keep going if left unchecked. The consequences from the behaviour and the growth opportunities afforded in letting go of the behaviour (boxes 2 and 3) are usually the most obvious to people, and often things that they think about all the time. Realistically, though, these are not the greatest motivators for change. In order to pursue change, people have to face the fantasy scripts they are holding on to (Box 1) as well as the fear they are experiencing in considering change (Box 4). It is also helpful to answer the questions below with each behaviour or substance you are looking to change.

What do I perceive I get out of using this behaviour or substance?

_____

_____

_____

_____

_____

What scripts, or stories, does my mind create about my use and engagement with this behaviour? (For example, that it is so much fun to drink heavily on Friday and Saturday nights; that I get so much relief from hiring an escort; that pornography has not impacted my sexual relationships).

_____

_____

_____

_____
_____
_____
_____

Are these stories based in reality?

_____
_____
_____
_____

What am I afraid of in considering changing this behaviour?

_____
_____
_____
_____
_____

It takes 2-5 years of action to get into the maintenance stage, where new behaviours feel more familiar and comfortable. It is important to appreciate that backsliding into contemplation can happen, so benefits and challenges need to be explored on an ongoing basis, in context of feelings.

ADDICTION INVOLVING RELATIONSHIPS

As you have been learning, Addiction can impact all aspects of life and behaviour to some extent. The impact on substance use and overtly destructive behaviours, especially ones that are life threatening, tend to overshadow the impact of Addiction on other areas of life, including relationships. However, it is important to keep in mind that Addiction lives in the part of the brain that controls our basic drive for survival: the reward circuitry. Therefore, it is likely that the behaviours rooted in this circuitry, primarily food, sex, love, and relationships will be implicated in Addiction. This part of the chapter is designed to help expand your awareness of how the disease may be impacting your social being. It is important to appreciate that in psychiatric terminology, this aspect of Addiction is often labelled 'Borderline Personality Disorder', which is often not helpful from a treatment or recovery perspective as it misses the other symptoms and manifestations of the disease.

List the challenges that tend to come up for you in relationships (romantic and otherwise). For example: conflict, avoiding issues, substance use, people not listening to you, abuse, secret-keeping, manipulation, difficulty with monogamy.

_____
_____
_____

_____
_____
_____
_____

List the strengths of your relationships (romantic and otherwise). For example: respect, calmness, openness, time to focus on your own health, understanding, reciprocity.

_____
_____
_____
_____
_____
_____
_____

Have you ever been caught off guard by a relationship suddenly ending or a major conflict arising? Write about that situation(s) – what happened and how it felt.

_____
_____
_____
_____
_____
_____
_____

How did you respond and cope with this surprise in the relationship?

_____
_____
_____
_____
_____

Relationships are where the 'D' and 'E' symptoms of Addiction often arise. These refer to: diminished recognition of problems in relationships and behaviour (D) and dysfunctional emotional response (E). These are the lifelong, or chronic, parts of the disease that will continue even after substance use or problematic behaviours are stable. If you have had multiple incidences of being caught off guard in relationships, this may be evidence of the 'D' of the disease; difficulty seeing the problems until it is too late. You may also have found yourself reacting inappropriately (either too much or too little) to situations, which is more indicative of the 'E' part of the disease impacting relationships. A helpful tool to keep exploring how your disease may be impacting relationships is the Karpman Triangle.

Karpman Triangle. Before we explain this concept in more detail, let us continue to explore how relationships have looked and felt in your life to date. We recommend completing this self-test using pencil or on a separate piece of paper so that you can return to it and track change over time.

Self-test: Place a check mark beside each statement that applies to you.

☐ 1. *I feel like people are out to purposefully hurt me*

☐ 2. *People take advantage of my good nature*

☐ 3. *Life has been very hard on me*

☐ 4. *Bad things seem to happen to me more than others I know*

☐ 5. *Life would be better if the people around me would change*

☐ 6. *I enjoy telling my friends and family about everything that is happening to me in my life*

☐ 7. *People are mean, bullying, and abusive towards me*

☐ 8. *I am uncomfortable with conflict*

☐ 9. *I prefer to keep my feelings to myself rather than express them*

☐ 10. *Life is not fair*

☐ 11. *I enjoy confrontation and conflict*

☐ 12. *I feel comfortable arguing with others*

☐ 13. *I have used physical force during conflict with others*

☐ 14. *I often raise my voice during arguments*

☐ 15. *I get mad and aggressive when people do not understand me*

☐ 16. *People who are passive frustrate me*

☐ 17. *The most common feelings for me are anger, frustration, and annoyance*

☐ 18. *People need to see things my way*

☐ 19. *I have provided money to people to bail them out of difficult situations*

☐ 20. *I am very concerned about the lives and well-being of others*

☐ 21. *I am one of the first people there to provide support to someone in need*

☐ 22. *I believe that my support of others is unconditional*

☐ 23. *I am so confused on what my needs and preferences are because I focus so much on what others want*

☐ 24. *I struggle with low self-esteem*

☐ 25. *I carry a lot of shame within me*

☐ 26. *My relationships are lacking emotional and/or physical intimacy and are quite superficial*

☐ 27. *Some of my behaviours feel unmanageable and are out of control*

☐ 28. *My emotional responses are either overreactions or under reactions to what the situation calls for*

This self-test is designed to give you some insight as to where you are on the Karpman Triangle.

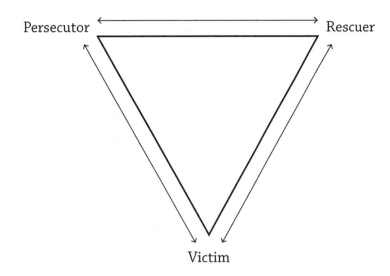

The Karpman Drama Triangle is a tool that was designed to illustrate the common roles in theatrical productions but can also refer to the roles people in unhealthy relationships take on. It is very likely that someone with Addiction will exhibit one, two, or all three of these roles at any given time. As people embrace recovery, they tend to move away from these roles and into healthier ones.

Now add up your checkmarks on the test and write down the totals:
Items 1–10:___ Items 11–18:___ Items 19–23:___ Items 24–28:___

Whatever columns you had the highest scores in indicate where you are most vulnerable on the Karpman Triangle. If you had the highest score on items 1–10, you are vulnerable of falling into the role of victim. People in the victim role tend to feel like life is happening to them and that they are unable to influence what is going on around them (helpless rather than powerless). This may lead them to be angry and blame the world (which can feed into perpetrator behaviours) and/or they may ruminate and get caught in feeling bad for themselves and their life. "Self pity" is often a term used for those stuck in the victim role.

Items 11–18 are indicative of the persecutor role. Persecutors tend to carry a lot of anger and resentment that spills out onto the world around them. Road rage, being irritable, arguments, propensity towards conflict, and having difficulty relaxing all tend to be frequent experiences for the perpetrator, who may or not physically act out towards others.

Items 19–23 comprise the experiences of the rescuer who is there to help people out at the expense of themselves. The rescuer is often enabling dysfunction in people around them, though believes they are doing good and 'helping' rather than hindering. The rescuer tends to neglect their own needs and desires for others.

If you did not identify with any or many of the statements up until items 24–28 but did have some checkmarks there, then chances are you may struggle with Addiction, as that is what these questions are highlighting. If you have Addiction, then likely at some points in your life you have found yourself acting within the Karpman Triangle as victim, persecutor, and/or rescuer but your blind pane may be so strong that you are having difficulty seeing this. If you don't identify with any of the roles, you are either engaging in healthy relationships or may have some avoidance of reality or denial.

As you move forward in recovery, we would encourage you to come back to this checklist periodically and redo it. As your level of awareness changes, your responses will also change and you may begin to see the patterns of disease in your relational interactions.

If you found yourself with high scores in multiple categories, that is not uncommon as people often take on multiple roles depending on the person they are interacting with and/or the situation. It is quite easy for the victim, who is internally feeling resentful, used, and abused to suddenly lash out and become the persecutor. The rescuer may slide into victim and/or persecutor particularly if they are not feeling listened to and do not have the control they are looking for.

As you look at these roles in your life, reflect on:

What is the motivation for my behaviour when I am in these roles?

_____
_____
_____
_____
_____

How am I feeling when I find myself in any of these roles?

_____
_____
_____
_____
_____

What am I really upset about when I am victim, persecutor, and rescuer? In other words, what is the real issue here?

_____
_____
_____
_____
_____

Looking honestly at these questions, while engaging in the pursuit of abstinence and holistic recovery, can help you move into the Recovery Roles triangle of helper, protector, and survivor. This triangle is pictured below.

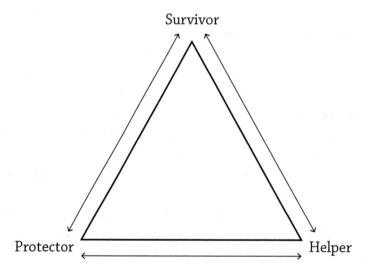

Self-test: Place a checkmark beside all the statements that apply to you.

☐ 1. *I share my feelings and concerns with others with no expectation of change*

☐ 2. *When offering advice, I do so with no attachment to outcome – I understand that others may accept my suggestions or they may not*

☐ 3. *My helping of others does not take away from my own life or self-care*

☐ 4. *I only offer what I can when supporting others, including financial assistance*

☐ 5. *I stop and consider my own feelings and needs before agreeing to help someone*

☐ 6. *The most important relationships in my life are with myself and my spirituality*

☐ 7. *I feel my relationships are reciprocal; there is mutual give and take*

☐ 8. *I feel respected, loved, and cared for in my relationships*

☐ 9. *I can be assertive in standing up for myself*

☐ 10. *I hold my loved ones accountable for their actions*

☐ 11. *I am there to offer support if asked, I do not force it upon anyone*

☐ 12. *I can enforce my own boundaries and know when they are being violated*

☐ 13. *I use consequences to reinforce accountability with others*

☐ 14. *I am gentle but firm in my approach with a struggling loved one*

☐ 15. *I use 'I' language in expressing feelings and thoughts*

☐ 16. *If I am feeling angry or upset, I take time to sit with, reflect, and process my feelings and thoughts before reacting*

☐ 17. *I feel empowered in my life*

☐ 18. *I know I have the ability to look after myself*

☐ 19. *I am responsible for my own health and well-being, first and foremost*

☐ 20. *I take time for self-care – looking after my physical, emotional, relational, and spiritual health*

☐ 21. *I take time to do fun activities that are healthy and nurturing for me*

☐ 22. *I look at my role in contributing to conflict or discord in relationships*

☐ 23. *I take accountability and own up to mistakes I have made*

☐ 24. *I am not defined by things that have happened in my past*

☐ 25. *I am open to processing issues, past and present, with an open mind*

☐ 26. *I am comfortable spending time with myself*

☐ 27. *I enjoy my relationships*

☐ 28. *I feel safe and at ease in my relationships*

For any of these boxes you have checked – Congratulations! This is information that you have been doing some valuable work in moving towards healthy, balanced relationships with self and others and are likely finding yourself in the recovery roles of helper, protector, and survivor. If you found that there were few or no checkmarks on the items above, then that is valuable information for you about where you are at in your recovery involving relationships. Likely you would benefit from the pursuit of abstinence from mood-altering substances and medications, as well as taking care of yourself differently in the areas of physical, emotional, social, and spiritual health. Each of these actions moves you closer towards being a helper, protector, and survivor.

What does it mean to you to be a helper in relationships rather than a rescuer?

_____

_____

_____

_____

_____

What does it mean to you to be a protector in relationships rather than a persecutor?

_____

_____

_____

_____

_____

What does it mean to you to be a survivor in relationships rather than a victim?

_____

_____

_____

_____

_____

How does it feel as you move from the Karpman Drama Triangle roles to the Recovery Roles triangle?

_____

_____

_____

_____

_____

Now would be a valuable time to look more closely at the relationships in your life and see how healthy the people around you are for your recovery. Complete the relationship map below to start exploring.

Make a list of all the people who are currently in your life. Leave space beside each name for additional writing. You can do this activity on a separate piece of paper, if needed.

Family:

_____

_____

_____

_____

_____

Friends:

_____

_____

_____

_____

_____

Acquaintances:

_____

_____

_____

_____

_____

Professional supports (doctors, psychologists, physiotherapists, etc.):

_____

_____

_____

_____

_____

Go back and beside each of these names, write down what role(s) you tend to take on with that person: Victim, persecutor, rescuer, helper, protector, or survivor.

Review your list and the roles you take on for each person. How do you feel about what you wrote down?

_____

_____

_____

_____

_____

What information does your list give you?

_____

_____

_____

_____

_____

For relationships where you acted as victim, persecutor, or rescuer, how could you move towards the recovery roles of helper, protector, and survivor?

_____

_____

_____

_____

_____

_____

_____

Is there anyone in your life currently that you may not be able to continue having a relationship with?

_____

_____

_____

_____

_____

How does this feel for you?

_____

_____

_____

_____

_____

How ready are you for action? Circle where you are at:

Very ready – let's do it   Hesitant, uncertain, doubting   Not ready at all

If you recognize that there may be a person or people in your life who are not contributing to your recovery but you are unsure if or when you may be able to set different boundaries with them, we would encourage you to keep talking with support people (not the person or people who you are struggling with) as well as journaling the feelings, reflections, memories, and experiences that come up or have been there in the past. It is only through this active processing that more awareness and clarity of what steps need to be taken will come. Perhaps in processing you become clearer on your needs, can be assertive and implement boundaries, and the relationship becomes healthier. Perhaps in processing you become clearer on your needs, can be assertive and implement boundaries, and the relationship stays the same or gets worse. Both of these are valuable scenarios because they give you the information needed to move to a greater readiness to change. Lots of feelings will come up along the way and they need to be felt and processed.

What fears come up when you consider looking at your relationships?

_____

_____

_____

_____

_____

What can you do for self-care to support yourself as you look at these relationships?

_____

_____

_____
_____
_____

"Stagnancy in recovery is never helpful and can lead to the disease taking back over again."

Looking honestly at relationships is probably the most difficult, yet most rewarding, part of recovery. It is only when people have explored this aspect of their life in the context of recovery that they continue to move forward to greater places of peace, love, and contentment, as well as overall happiness. Many shy away from looking at relationships in their recovery and focus just on maintaining abstinence from substances or behaviours. If this is you, we would gently remind you that you are missing out on a valuable opportunity for growth. Stagnancy in recovery is never helpful and can lead to the disease taking back over again. Next, we cover some other things to consider as you move forward with behaviour change, both within and outside of relationships.

STRATEGIES FOR BEHAVIOUR CHANGE

We hear often that recovery feels overwhelming, daunting, and is hard work. We also hear that recovery is incredibly rewarding, uplifting, and gratifying. Both of these are accurate, but if you have yet to experience the benefits of recovery, that can make it hard to keep moving forward through the uncomfortable parts. Here is an opportunity to look at gratitude and the gifts of recovery.

List all of the gifts you have received in your ongoing pursuit of recovery (e.g., new relationships, Higher Power moments, accomplishments, feelings, physical health improvements):

_____
_____
_____
_____
_____

What are the biggest barriers for you in pursuing recovery?

_____
_____
_____
_____
_____

Often when people are reflecting on barriers (in addition to the obvious one of having the chronic disease of Addiction), the challenges tend to fall into one of three categories: Environment, exposure, and stress. This is the language used by the ASAM definition of Addiction and is an off-shoot of the 12-Step language of 'people, places, and things.' What both of these lists are referring to are the triggers, or activators, of the disease that can interfere with recovery motivation and progress. Let us explore what these look like in your life in more depth.

Environment. The brain reacts to being in familiar environments, including those associated with active Addiction, in mere milliseconds, which is not even enough time for us to consciously be aware of the impact these places are having on us. However, with awareness of this brain vulnerability and some processing, people can develop a fairly clear sense of environments that are supportive of recovery for them. In doing this, it will also be obvious what environments, or places, are not.

Write down the environments (places) where you feel safe, comfortable, at ease, calm, or serene. If you cannot identify any of these places right now, write down the places where you feel somewhat comfortable. Usually these environments will not involve your substance or behaviour of most effective reward, relief or escape being present.

_____

_____

_____

_____

_____

_____

_____

Write down more about how you feel when you are in these environments.

_____

_____

_____

_____

_____

_____

_____

What is it about these environments that are supportive of your recovery?

_____

_____

_____

_____

_____

It is also important to be honest about the environments you might be finding yourself in that are aggravating of the disease, or triggering.

What environments do you feel uncomfortable, out of place, withdrawn, isolated, down, or activated in?

_____

_____

_____

_____

_____

Write down more about how you feel when you are in these places.

_____

_____

_____

_____

_____

What features of these environments do not support your recovery?

_____

_____

_____

_____

_____

Often environments that feel activating and triggering involve some exposure to substances or problem behaviours. These may not necessarily have been your main substances or behaviours but the disease still finds them enticing. For example, being in a pub even though you primarily drank at home or being at a party with a junk food and treat buffet even though you have not identified food as a primary challenge for you. Let us explore further the role of exposure to substance and behaviour in your life.

What substances and problem behaviours are your main challenges?

_____

_____

_____

_____

_____

Where do you get exposed to these substances and behaviours?

_____

_____

_____

_____

_____

What people expose you to these substances and behaviours?

_____

_____

_____

_____

_____

What can you do to minimize your exposure to these substances and behaviours? In other words, what is your action plan?

_____
_____
_____
_____
_____

Sometimes people may inadvertently find themselves in a situation that becomes uncomfortable and, no matter how much planning or forethought went into it, they could not have prevented this exposure from happening. For example, someone shows up with marijuana to a sober event; people smoking cigarettes outside of a 12-Step meeting; or people drinking alcohol at a child's birthday party. When you are planning on going out to events and social gatherings, it is important to always have a safety plan and exit strategy in mind. Let us work on creating yours now.

If you found yourself in an uncomfortable situation, what would you do to keep yourself safe?

_____
_____
_____
_____
_____

Who can you call for support?

_____
_____
_____
_____
_____

Where can you go in that setting that is safer (e.g., with different people, different room)?

_____
_____
_____
_____
_____

When can you leave and how?

_____
_____
_____
_____
_____

If you are with someone, can you have a code word that signifies, "I need to leave now"?

Write that code word down here:

If you are planning a trip, whether for leisure or work, it is also important to have a recovery plan and exit strategy for that as well.

What is your self-care plan when you are away? Can you put these activities into your calendar?

_____
_____
_____
_____
_____

Who will you contact for support during the trip?

_____
_____
_____
_____
_____

Will there be exposure to substances and problem behaviours on the trip that are known?

_____
_____
_____
_____
_____

What can you do to minimize this exposure?

_____
_____
_____
_____
_____

Where can you go if you are uncomfortable?

_____
_____
_____
_____
_____

Can you give yourself permission to cut the trip short if needed?

_____

How are you feeling about the upcoming trip?

_____
_____
_____

_____

_____

What do these feelings tell you about the trip?

_____

_____

_____

_____

_____

If you do not have any travel booked in the near future, these are helpful questions to come back to for planning before you do. They are even more helpful to consider before *booking* a trip so that, if needed, you can adjust your plan accordingly and hopefully not find yourself in a disease activating situation. Travel is challenging for recovery as it throws off the routine and structure that has been established so it is essential that some recovery routine is maintained while away. Twelve-Step meetings, journaling, meditation, physical activity, and peer support via phone, Skype, text, or e-mail are the most common tools that are travel-friendly.

Exposure to substances and problem behaviours is very activating for the brain, just like environment and feelings of stress. When we are stressed, we have higher amounts of cortisol, adrenaline, and norepinephrine released in the body, which makes us more reactive. With Addiction being a disease of escape, relief, and reward, an increased amount of stress can make one vulnerable to wanting to seek escape or relief from that activation in unhealthy ways. Likewise, when people are in an acutely stressful situation that ends, they may feel the desire to reward themselves using substances or problem behaviours that are unmanageable or become so over time. It is important to be aware of your vulnerabilities with stress and to have a plan of action for self-care to counteract its potentially triggering impact.

Make a list of your top 10 most stressful events and situations:

1.

2.

3.

4.

5.

6.

7.

8.

9.

10.

What are your typical ways of coping with these stressful events? List them all here.

_____
_____
_____
_____
_____
_____
_____

Beside each item above, label whether you would deem them healthy (H) or unhealthy (U) ways of coping.

What are some additional healthy methods of coping that you have not tried, would like to try, or think you have tried that have not worked? Write them all down here.

_____
_____
_____
_____
_____

Which of the strategies in the previous question are you willing to start (re)incorporating into your self-care routine to help you deal with stress? List them here.

_____
_____
_____
_____
_____

Now be specific about how and when you are going to incorporate these into your routine. For example, what time of day, for how long, and with whom (if applicable).

_____
_____
_____
_____
_____

_____
_____

What barriers do you foresee coming up in bringing these into your routine?

_____
_____
_____
_____
_____

For the methods of coping you wrote down that you had tried before that had not worked, elaborate on what seemed ineffective about them.

_____
_____
_____
_____
_____

For these self-care items that you have deemed 'did not work,' we would encourage you to consider trying them again. It is always amazing the resistance the brain may have to certain ideas at certain times. At other times, the brain may be very open and you may find great benefit in the same tool(s). Often it is not the tools that are the issue, it is the level of openness (or lack thereof) that gets in the way.

What self-care strategy(ies) are you willing to try adding to your ritual again?

_____
_____
_____
_____
_____

"Give yourself at least three weeks of regularly incorporating this tool into your routine..."

Give yourself at least three weeks of regularly incorporating this tool into your routine before you make a fair assessment of its utility. It takes quite some time to get used to things and for them to have a visible benefit. Doing something once or twice is not going to be a realistic gauge of its effectiveness. After trying out the strategy for three weeks, take some time to journal about your feelings and ask for feedback from others on any changes they have noticed in you to see if this is something you wish to continue as part of your self-care routine.

As was discussed in *Addiction is Addiction* and the chapter in this workbook on addictive thinking, self-talk can be a powerful way of coaching ourselves through difficult moments, including ones that are intensely stressful. We can use calming statements, reality checks, and affirmations to help lower stress levels and ground us in the here and now.

List five calming phrases, words, or statements you could repeat to yourself when you are feeling stressed (e.g., 'Relax. Breathe in, out' or 'This too shall pass'):

1.

2.

3.

4.

5.

List five phrases or statements that bring you back to reality (e.g., 'This feeling and situation will change as all the rest have done before,' or 'I can handle all of my feelings'):

1.

2.

3.

4.

5.

List five affirmations of strengths you possess that will help you deal with times of stress (e.g., 'I am capable of getting through this,' or 'I can handle what life throws my way'):

1.

2.

3.

4.

5.

Once you have these statements, you can build on them over time by incorporating more affirmations and developing phrases that counteract addictive thinking statements. For example, rather than allowing your brain to carry on with the thought of "I can't do this, this is hard," you may shift that to, "I can handle this moment and the next and the next. I am capable." Once you have some of these statements and affirmations, we would recommend that you bring them into consciousness regularly throughout the day.

Pick one phrase from the list above and repeat it multiple times on at least three separate occasions throughout the day (out loud or in your head).

Realistic self-talk, in addition to being aware of other triggers and having an ongoing self-care routine, are essential for helping reduce vulnerability to environment, exposure, and stress. Here are some additional steps for incorporating behaviour change into your life:

- *Take it slow – focus on one priority step at a time*

- *Reduce goals by at least half (e.g., if your brain says to exercise for 40 minutes/day, four times/week, do it 20 minutes/day for two times/week)*

- *Be realistic in your goals for yourself, both in terms of outcome and the path to get there*

- *Pick somewhere to start, even if it seems small (e.g., drinking more water in a day). All change leads to change*

- *Remember it is about progress, not perfection*

- *Everyone's pace is different. Follow your pace, not others*

- *Give yourself at least three weeks of regular practice before you start evaluating whether something is working or not. Change takes time*

- *Be open about your desires with others in order to foster accountability*

- *Be honest about the challenges that are coming up as you look to change*

- *Focus on gratitude and growth, not judgement and shame*

Change takes time but does happen slowly but surely so the key is to start somewhere and focus on your goals, not expectations for what will happen if you engage in change. The path of change will likely unfold very differently from what your mind created, but that is not a bad thing. In fact, that is the beauty of recovery and trusting the process: you always get what you need, although it may not always be what you want (or thought you wanted).

Key messages

- Addiction can manifest in many substances and behaviours.

- The disease can manifest in all aspects of life; the key to recovery is being able to recognize the disease influence and work on choosing recovery.

- Many people new to recovery worry that looking at all of these different aspects of their lives will make life 'not fun' anymore, which is not what recovery is about at all.

- Yes, it can be hard work and uncomfortable at times, but recovery enables you to connect with true fun and self and enjoy a better quality of life.

Action steps for Chapter 5 (follow through after chapter exercises)

There were many different focuses throughout this chapter but a major one was on relationships. Moving forward, we would encourage you to keep learning about healthy communication, assertiveness, boundaries, and addressing relationship challenges in your life as these will pose barriers to your recovery. This can be through additional reading, workshops, talking with recovery supports, step work, volunteer and service work, introspection, and practice.

Chapter 6: Holistic Recovery: A Bio-Psycho-Social-Spiritual Perspective

'New beginnings are often disguised as painful endings.'
—Lao Tzu

What does recovery mean to you?

_____

_____

_____

_____

_____

Recovery is available to everyone, including those who do not have Addiction. Recovery is about living an authentic, healthy, balanced life and having the opportunity to become the best version of you. Recovery is a process that can fuel fear, vulnerability, and angst. However, it can also propel freedom, serenity, relief, connection, and authenticity. In this chapter we will explore the important components of recovery, its relationship with behaviour, and treatment from a holistic perspective.

RECOVERY IS …

- *The continued pursuit of health and personal growth*

- ***It is NOT**: magic, a quick-fix, a cure*

- ***It IS**: lifestyle, a process, slowly shifting the focus to health and wellness in all areas (biological, psychological, social, and spiritual)*

What are your challenges to recovery action at this time?

☐ No time

☐ Lack of support from others

☐ Too much pressure from others

☐ Weather (e.g., too cold, too hot)

☐ Lack of money

☐ Disease activity

☐ Rationalization

☐ Minimization

☐ Belief that: "It's not working"

☐ Feeling disconnected

☐ Desire to isolate

☐ Work

☐ Family, kids

☐ Feeling okay

☐ Too tired, no energy

☐ Lack of motivation

☐ Don't see a problem

☐ Just don't want to

☐ Other(s): _____

The biggest challenge to recovery is LIFE.

Recovery into life means:

- *Life continues to take priority over recovery*

- *Recovery action is fit around the daily tasks and priorities of life (work, kids, chores, bills, events, etc.)*

- *This is not a viable plan as life will overtake recovery, allowing disease activity to increase*

- *Recovery action diminishes over time*

For optimal recovery, it becomes life into recovery:

- *This requires faith and trust that things will work out as they need to, not necessarily as you want or expect them to*

- *Rather than trying to control life, be accountable to recovery*

- *Build a recovery lifestyle that other aspects of life rotate around, not vice versa*

COMPONENTS OF RECOVERY

Self-management combined with mutual support is important in recovery from Addiction. Mutual support, such as that found in community-based 12-Step groups (Alcoholics Anonymous, Narcotics Anonymous, etc.) is beneficial as it touches on the emotional, social, and spiritual aspects of recovery. Recovery from Addiction is best achieved through a combination of self-management, mutual support, and professional care provided by trained and certified professionals.

"... the emphasis needs to be on structure and discipline, not control, which can feed the disease."

Self-management. These are the strategies that an individual can use for themselves to improve health along the bio-psycho-social-spiritual dimensions of health. Some examples include maintaining a healthy and balanced diet, getting adequate sleep, regular exercise, managing daily responsibilities, finding time for fun activities, talking, sharing, developing and maintaining a spiritual connection. There are numerous options available in each category and recovery will require some exploration of different strategies to see which ones are best suited to you at this particular time. Self-management tools may change over time as you evolve in yourself and recovery. We are using the term self-management as it is a commonly used one but the emphasis needs to be on structure and discipline, not control, which can feed the disease.

What self-management strategies have you used in your recovery to date?

_____
_____
_____
_____
_____

What self-management strategies would you like to try?

_____
_____
_____
_____
_____

What have been the barriers to taking action with these strategies?

_____
_____

_____

_____

_____

Mutual support. Mutual (or peer) support is essential for long-term recovery. Mutual support can come from existing friends or family but often there are challenges to this. Sometimes existing friends or family members are old 'using buddies', so even being around these individuals, particularly in early recovery, can increase vulnerability and risk of relapse. Sometimes existing friends or family members may be unhealthy themselves and struggle with the same disease of Addiction that may or may not be acknowledged. In a lot of instances, the support that the person entering recovery may want or need will not be available from these existing 'supports'. Thus, mutual support coming from new friends, namely others in recovery, is a healthier option.

The benefit of surrounding oneself with peers in recovery is powerful. These are people you can personally relate to and who are working on being authentic themselves. Peers in recovery can provide the support, experience, and wisdom that others who are not in recovery may be unable to provide. Like all new friendships, building recovery supports takes time and effort so it is important to give yourself the time to build these new connections.

Who is part of your peer support circle?

_____

_____

_____

_____

_____

What have you heard from your peer support circle that feels loving and joyous to you?

_____

_____

_____

_____

_____

12-Step Programs. Alcoholics Anonymous (AA) is the original 12-Step program, founded in 1935 by Mr. Bill Wilson and Dr. Robert Smith. Addiction was perceived rather narrowly at the time as alcoholism, usually considered a weakness, character flaw or moral failing that defied cure. There were limited treatment options available to those struggling, hence the creation of AA, as a mutual support program. While Addiction was primarily perceived as a personal failing and choice, there were those at the time, including one of Bill W.'s treating physicians, Dr. William Silkworth, who believed it was more than that. Dr. Silkworth believed that alcoholism was a disease that came with 'obsession' of the mind and a physical 'allergy' of the body, which manifested as craving for more alcohol.

In today's world, we have come to appreciate that allergies involve the immune system and are a defensive response towards specific antigens that the body perceives as toxic. As much as alcohol and other substances of abuse may be toxic to the body, the immune system is not engaged. Dr. Silkworth emphasized that alcoholism was a disease, rather than people making bad choices. In addition to his theory about alcoholism, Dr. Silkworth also indicated that abstinence was necessary in order for recovery to be possible. We have come to appreciate that the 'obsession' of the mind is actually craving for relief. The 'allergy' of the body is intensification of that craving after consuming the substance. This is the trigger for 'more' that arises out of activation of the brain circuits associated with Addiction even with exposure to small amounts of addictive substances such as opioids (in pain medication), depressants (in anti-anxiety or sleep medications) and small amounts of alcohol present in 'de-alcoholized' beer or wine or 'near beer'.

How familiar are you with the history of AA? How do you feel about what you are reading here?

_____

_____

_____

_____

_____

The involvement of memory circuits with Addiction means that even the appearance (visual), smell, sounds, touch, and/or taste associated with addictive products from one's past can trigger craving.

In recovery, list the substances or behaviours that you find triggering, that bring about cravings, and/or feel unsettling for you to be around:

_____

_____

_____

_____

_____

What are your sensory triggers?

Sight/visual:

_____

_____

_____

_____

Smells:

_____

_____

_____

_____

Sounds:

_____

_____

_____

_____

Touch:

_____

_____

_____

_____

_____

Tastes:

_____

_____

_____

_____

_____

Although Bill W. spent time with a Christian fellowship called the Oxford Group, he realized that religion could be a barrier to recovery, hence, the creation of a concept of a higher power that people could define more personally. It is important to appreciate that religion was specifically left out of *The Big Book* and spirituality was emphasized instead. Religion can be a means for spirituality for those that connect with it but it is not necessary for spirituality, which is a more personal connection with one's self and the rest of the universe.

What is your personal understanding of the distinction between spirituality and religion?

_____

_____

_____

_____

_____

Since the inception of AA in 1935, the 12-Step fellowship has blossomed around the world and developed groups that focus on substances or behaviours in addition to alcohol, including narcotics (NA); gambling (GA); overeating (OA); code-pendency (CoDA); sex and love (SA, SAA, SLAA); anorexia and bulimia (ABA); and emotions (EA). There are also groups for family members of people with Addiction, such as Al-Anon, Nar-Anon, and Gam-Anon.

All of these programs are free, community based, volunteer led and managed, and available all around the world. While 12-Step groups are not sufficient for the entirety of treatment for people struggling with Addiction (meaning additional tools, groups, treatment, or resources are usually necessary), they are certainly a valuable resource that is available most places at most times, making it one of the most accessible recovery options in the world.

Many people struggle with the idea of attending these programs, particularly if they have not been to one before or have preconceived notions about it, including the spirituality aspect. While many describe these groups as religious, this is a fallacy. The 12-Step programs contain valuable spiritual principles within them that transcend religious belief. Addiction is an isolating disease, so the steps are designed to have one look beyond one's self and connect with something greater. This can be nature, other people, the universe, energy, the solar system, or anything you understand it to be; it does not have to be God. Some people refer to GOD as Good Orderly Direction, providing structure and discipline. The AA concept of 'God of one's own understanding' is areligious and is actually considered blasphemous by some Christian groups.

How would you describe your current spiritual belief system?

_____

_____

_____

_____

_____

What feelings does discussion of spirituality bring up for you?

_____

_____

_____

_____

_____

From a holistic recovery perspective, the process of mutual support available in 12-Step meetings provides growth in the emotional-social-spiritual realms.

From your perspective or experience, what benefits do 12-Step meetings provide for:

Emotional health:

_____

_____

_____

_____

_____

Social health:

_____

_____

_____

_____

_____

Spiritual health:

_____

_____

_____

_____

_____

From an emotional perspective, 12-step programs allow one to explore what it means to have a primary, chronic disease; the implications and consequence of the disease on self and others; the character traits that need to be worked on for a healthy self; and having a place (whether in meetings, reaching out to people in the program or working individually with a sponsor) to talk openly about feelings and experiences with people who understand. You cannot put a price on the value of feeling heard and being understood, in the context of seeking clarity oneself.

Socially, these meetings allow people to connect with other people who have Addiction, or have been impacted by Addiction and are in recovery. This can feel much safer than associating with people who are active in their Addiction or do not understand the disease at all. This does not mean your social network will be free of people in active Addiction but it's an opportunity to turn to people who also have the disease and are in recovery.

Finally, spiritually, there is immense opportunity within the 12-Step program to explore yourself, your internal spirit, and self-worth, and begin reaching out to others through living amends and service work.

What do you think of 12-Step meetings?

_____

_____

_____

_____

_____

What works for you at meetings?

_____

_____

_____

_____

_____

What does not work for you at meetings?

_____

_____

_____

_____

_____

If you have not attended a 12-Step meeting, what are the barriers to attending?

_____

_____

_____

_____

_____

If you have not attended a 12-Step meeting, what would it take to get you to try it?

_____

_____

_____

_____

_____

Professional support. It is important to find a healthcare provider, or team of practitioners, who are educated and knowledgeable about the disease of Addiction and can support the person in recovery through the holistic process of recovery. Objective outsiders are able to hear the disease in action more clearly than the addicted mind, so even peer supports can at times get trapped by the allure and seeming logic of addictive thinking.

What professional support do you have?

_____
_____
_____
_____
_____

Is it meeting your needs? If yes, what is working for you? If no, what are you missing? If a combination, identify what is working and where the gaps are.

_____
_____
_____
_____
_____

How satisfied are you with your current recovery?

1-------2-------3-------4-------5-------6-------7-------8-------9-------10

Dissatisfied   Somewhat satisfied   Very Satisfied

Wherever you are on the scale above, there is always room for growth in the realm of self-exploration and if you stop moving forward in recovery, you will get pulled back down into disease. In the next section we start exploring more specific strategies you can use to continue your recovery using a holistic approach to health.

BIO-PSYCHO-SOCIAL-SPIRITUAL (HOLISTIC) RECOVERY

Individuals with Addiction entering recovery have come to a place of realization that what they are doing is no longer working for them. Some have hit their rock bottom. Others have not had tremendous consequence from their Addiction but recognize the unmanageability and powerlessness of the disease. Drugs are now ingested because they 'have to', not because they are wanted or desired; hours spent on the casino floor now feel dreadful; and the physical, emotional, and relational highs and lows of the Addiction have become tortuous.

Describe your 'rock bottom' or turning point of change. How did you know it was time to do something different in your life?

_____
_____

_____
_____
_____

How did you feel at this time?

_____
_____
_____
_____
_____

As Addiction has been the reality for so long, the process and promises of recovery can seem unattainable, daunting, and unfamiliar. Sometimes fear of the known feels less scary than the fear of the unknown, hence the saying "better the devil you know than the devil you don't". Through education, time, awareness, and action, the unique process of recovery will begin to unfold at the levels of: attention to physical health (biological) with healthy eating and exercise, clarifying thinking and feeling distortions with an emphasis on processing feelings (psychological), developing a new, supportive social network (social), and alignment of values and meaning in life (spiritual).

What has recovery action looked like for you, to date, in each of these categories?

Biological:

_____
_____
_____
_____

Psychological/emotional:

_____
_____
_____
_____

Social:

_____
_____
_____
_____

Spiritual:

_____
_____

Consider Addiction as a bio-psycho-social-spiritual disease with observable, wide-ranging behavioural manifestations. This is also a useful approach for recovery. Just as the disease of Addiction manifests differently in everyone, with some common traits and underpinnings, so the process of recovery unfolds in a unique and individualized way, with some basic underlying principles. Therefore, individuals learn to tailor their recovery program to themselves with a combination of help from professional treatment and non-professional mutual support.

It must be appreciated that *all* aspects of the disease need to be explored rather than focusing on just one substance or overt behaviour problem.

How does Bio-Psycho-Social-Spiritual (Holistic) recovery resonate with you? What do you agree with? What are you having trouble with?

_____

_____

_____

_____

_____

Biological. The biological, or physical, aspect of holistic recovery is the most accessible and familiar. When entering recovery, it is important to be thoroughly examined by a physician, preferably one who is experienced in Addiction Medicine. For many people with Addiction, it has been years since they have had a regular physical check-up because of fear and shame related to what complications may be developing. Having an examination can provide a starting point to see if regular medical care and treatment is necessary. If this is not done, the recovery work that one begins may be hampered by ongoing physical symptoms that have not been attended to. For example, pain from a physical health issue contributes to feelings of frustration and lack of energy. These feelings then become attributed to the process of recovery not working.

Other aspects of physical health include diet and exercise. Nutritionally valuable foods are important to consume, especially while the body is recalibrating without substance or problem behaviours to soothe itself. Hydration with water helps flush the system and eating regularly throughout the day stabilizes blood sugar and metabolic processes. Regular physical activity (20 minutes, 3–4 times per week as a general guideline) provides routine and structure to recovery in addition to the health benefits it provides, including lowered cholesterol, maintenance of healthy weight, muscle strengthening, and cardiovascular benefits. For those who are reluctant to engage in exercise, walking around the block or neighbourhood is a great place to start.

Biological recommendations

- *Regular exercise/physical activity (20–30 minutes/day, 3–4x/week) e.g., walking, cycling, yoga, cardio, weights, organized sports, swimming, gardening, Tai Chi.*

How often do you exercise and do physical activity?

_____

_____

_____

_____

_____

What physical activities do you enjoy?

_____

_____

_____

_____

_____

What other activities would benefit your physical health in recovery?

_____

_____

_____

_____

_____

If you are not doing regular (or any) exercise, what is holding you back?

_____

_____

_____

_____

_____

- *A healthy, balanced diet*

   A balanced diet is one that gives your body the nutrients it needs to function properly. If there are no food allergies or sensitivities, in order to get the proper nutrition from your diet, it is best to obtain the majority of your daily calories from fresh fruits and vegetables, whole grains, legumes, nuts, and lean proteins.

   Water is essential to good health, yet needs vary by individual. You may need to modify your total fluid intake depending on how active you are, the climate you live in, your health status, and if you are pregnant or breastfeeding.

Do you regularly have a healthy, balanced diet?

_____

_____

_____

_____

_____

What are your challenges in consistently pursuing healthy eating?

_____

_____

_____
_____
_____

What are three things you are willing and able to do to eat healthier?

1.

2.

3.

- *Healthy sleep patterns*

   Sleep is a vital indicator of overall health and well-being as we spend up to one-third of our lives asleep. Like diet and exercise, sleep is a critical component to overall health.

   Healthy sleep tips include sticking to a sleep schedule (even on weekends); practicing a relaxing bedtime ritual (e.g., journaling, meditation, reading, a bath); exercising regularly; evaluating your bedroom to ensure ideal temperature, sound, and light; sleeping on a comfortable mattress and pillows; considering sleeping on your own if your sleep mate (partner or pets) are disruptive; being aware of common chemicals that affect both quantity and quality of sleep such as caffeine, alcohol, nicotine, antihistamines as well as prescription medications including beta blockers, alpha blockers, and antidepressants; and turning off all electronics at least 30 minutes before bed.

How much sleep do you typically get a night?

_____
_____
_____
_____
_____

Do you feel well rested in the morning when you get up?

_____
_____
_____
_____
_____

What are your challenges in the realm of sleep?

_____
_____
_____
_____
_____

What three changes can you make to improve your sleep?

1.

2.

3.

Psychological/Emotional. The reality of 'feeling the feelings' can be daunting. After all, these are the feelings that the addictive process has escaped, avoided, and sought relief from. People get worried that once they start feeling the feelings that they will be unable to deal with them. Fear takes over and blocks the feelings from coming. It is important to appreciate that fear itself is just a feeling and will pass, just as all other feelings do. Feelings are valuable information and provide us with knowledge about ourselves and the people and situations around us. It is important not to deprive ourselves of this information as it is crucial for health.

> *"It is important to appreciate that fear is just a feeling and will pass, just as all other feelings do."*

As feelings arise, one can write about them, paint about them, talk about them, reflect on them, sit with them, emote about them, and explore them. Over time, the person in recovery will find their personal and unique ways to deal with feelings using a variety of techniques. The psychological aspect of recovery attends to feelings and brings in a focus on self-talk as well as paying attention to addictive thinking.

People often confuse the words empathy and sympathy. In recovery, it is important to focus on empathy, which means 'the ability to understand and share the feelings of another' whereas sympathy means 'feelings of pity and sorrow for someone else's misfortune'. The vulnerability with sympathy is taking on someone else's emotions, pain, and suffering as our own which fuels enmeshment and taking on other people's issues rather than staying 'on your side of the street'. Empathy reinforces healthy boundaries, allowing people to still care, love, and support each other without rescuing and becoming part of the problem. It also provides the opportunity for the other person to figure out the solution to their own issues so they become a survivor, not a victim, as discussed in the previous chapter.

Can you give example of when you have been empathetic?

_____
_____
_____
_____
_____

Can you give examples of when you have been sympathetic?

_____
_____
_____

_____

_____

Psychological/Emotional recommendations

- *Focus on identifying and processing emotions e.g., journaling, talking, art*

- *Consider individual and/or group counselling, exploration of trauma, mental health and coping mechanisms e.g., relaxation, meditation, breathing*

- *Foster serenity by paying attention to the language within yourself: transform self-talk to be more accepting and compassionate, start incorporating a daily gratitude journal and identify three things you are grateful for each day*

- *Practice affirmations*

- *Talk with others to check out addictive thinking*

- *Self-care: doing fun, relaxing activities to balance recovery and life work, e.g., sports, cooking classes, baking, arts & crafts, games/puzzles, time with animals, going for walks*

- *'Play the tape through': Reflect on consequences of past use, not just benefit/relief/reward*

How do you typically deal with feelings?

_____

_____

_____

_____

_____

How are you feeling right now?

_____

_____

_____

_____

_____

Do you check in your thinking and feelings with others in recovery? If not, what are some of the barriers for you?

_____

_____

_____

_____

_____

What do you currently do for fun?

_____

_____

_____

_____

_____

List three things you consider fun that you are currently not doing and want to start or restart:

1.

2.

3.

List three things you are grateful for today:

1.

2.

3.

Practice affirmations. Name five things that you appreciate and value about yourself:

1.

2.

3.

4.

5.

Social. The social aspect of recovery revolves around relationships, old and new. Some people will naturally drift out of life, some will be actively detached from because they fuel vulnerability, and others will come into life as a gift of recovery. As the saying goes, "people come into your life for a reason, a season, or a lifetime."

As the mind clears in recovery, existing relationships often feel different. Take Anne, as an example. Anne had been a daily drinker for the past two years. She initially was able to drink in moderation with her husband and collecting wine and visiting wineries was a shared passion of theirs. As their children left home and she had more spare time, Anne found herself drinking during the day before her husband got home from work. When Anne decided to engage in the recovery process, her husband and family were supportive. They were hopeful that once she got treatment, she would someday be able to drink in moderation again. Initially, Anne found daily living, which included taking care of all the household chores, overwhelming and frustrating. Cleaning the house became a major stressor that she felt incapable of dealing with sober. She soon realized how lonely and isolated she had become and struggled with frequent relapses. After multiple relapses, Anne decided she needed to go away to residential treatment, where she could focus on her personal journey of recovery away from her home environment. When Anne's husband participated in the family portion of the program, she continued to struggle with assertiveness as she did not want to disappoint him or change his lifestyle in anyway. She struggled to figure out how she could be in recovery while her husband continued to drink wine. Over time, she learned to communicate assertively, set appropriate boundaries, and engage in self-care when feelings were coming up for her. Dealing with conflict and the possibility that others may get upset is particularly challenging in recovery, as this challenges the image management and relationship parts of the disease that call for civility regardless of what is happening and the desire to maintain peace at all costs.

How do you currently deal with conflict?

_____
_____
_____
_____
_____

How do these strategies work for you?

_____
_____
_____
_____
_____

How do these strategies not work for you?

_____
_____
_____
_____
_____

In recovery, the dysfunction or illness of extended family (parents, siblings, spouses, children) may become apparent. It is discomforting to see sickness in loved ones, as often they have been placed on a pedestal. We see them as ideal, not real. Families often create a dynamic in which the visibly active person with Addiction is the 'sick one' and everybody else is a witness, not an active participant in the disease. The focus is on the identified person and desperate calls for treatment and support are pushed toward this individual. This dynamic of 'us' and 'them' becomes routine in the family and when the identified 'problem' person begins to get well, this creates a significant shift for the others. Now attention and energy is freed up that allows family members to reflect on themselves and, more often than not, they realize that they have also been part of the problem. The feelings that arise from these realities are challenging, but also offer profound opportunities for growth.

How have your relationships with family changed since being in recovery?

_____
_____

_____
_____
_____

How have these changes felt for you?

_____
_____
_____
_____
_____

Reality shifts in recovery. More accurately, reality is not shifting so much as the *perception* of it. The people, places, and things the person in recovery thought they knew and understood changes as they gain clarity, and this is often where the appreciation of a need to make both minor and major changes in lifestyle arise.

Give some examples of how your perception has shifted in recovery:

_____
_____
_____
_____
_____
_____
_____

Adam, father of four, struggled with sobriety throughout his life. However, once he was able to maintain some clean time, he started to gain some clarity and realized that his eldest son was trapped in his own disease. This created drama and chaos in the house, increasing conflict between his wife and himself as they could not agree on how to deal with the situation. This made it extremely challenging for Adam to maintain his recovery action. Only when he was able to step back from these relationships, disconnect with love for a period of time, and focus on himself were the promises of recovery able to blossom in his life. This was Adam's challenge. For others it might be relationships, past trauma, shame, or the desire for control that are barriers to recovery. As one begins the process of recovery, the personal barriers will become clear, with the help of peer and professional support, and one will be able to devise a recovery plan that allows them to deal with these challenges in a healthy way.

Social recommendations

- *12-Step meetings or other community support groups*

- *Developing recovery peer supports*

- *Addressing relationship issues*

- *Work, school, volunteering*

- *Engagement with others to minimize isolation –"From isolation to connectedness ..."*

What social relationships were in your life when your disease was active?

_____
_____
_____

_____

_____

What social activities are feeding or enabling your disease?

_____

_____

_____

_____

_____

What social relationships are important in supporting your recovery?

_____

_____

_____

_____

_____

What social activities are helping your recovery?

_____

_____

_____

_____

_____

What relationship issues are you currently dealing with?

_____

_____

_____

_____

_____

"Spirituality is the discovery of our authentic self without any trimmings or labels."

Spiritual. The role of spirituality in recovery may be undermined or neglected by healthcare providers, treatment programs, as well as the individual pursuing recovery. Often spirituality becomes likened to or synonymous with religion, which is a sensitive topic for many people, particularly if they have been raised in a religious environment or have a challenging relationship with God, church, and religion. Spirituality is the discovery of our authentic self without any trimmings or labels. Spirituality gifts us with a rich source of values and a deeper meaning to life, whatever our religion may or may not be. Religion can be a means to an end in spirituality for those for whom that is important, but it is not a necessary means.

As previously discussed, spirituality connects the person with a love and force outside of themselves, being their Higher Power of choice. In recovery, feeling unconditional love and understanding that one is not alone are powerful antidotes to the feelings of abandonment, loneliness, self-hatred, and shame that stem from the disease of Addiction. Connecting with a HP through meditation, prayer, time in nature, reflection, reading, or journaling fosters a sense of serenity, peacefulness, and calm that can, in the early days of recovery, be helpful when cravings and uncomfortable feelings surface. As recovery progresses and this relationship strengthens, it becomes the foundation for long-term abstinence and leads to the promises of recovery.

How is your current relationship with your Higher Power?

_____
_____
_____
_____
_____

How are you able to connect with your Higher Power?

_____
_____
_____
_____
_____

How can your relationship with your Higher Power be strengthened further?

_____
_____
_____
_____
_____

"The recovery process is self-focused, not selfish."

Addiction is often described as a 'selfish' disease. Certainly when people are entrenched in it the focus is on self—more specifically, the disease's quest for escape, relief, and reward through substance or problem behaviours. Even recovery can be (mis)perceived as selfish, but more accurately, the recovery process is *self-focused*, not selfish. A gift of recovery is the ability to share one's love and personal attributes with others because life is no longer driven by one's own pleasure, but rather pleasure in all the things life has to offer, including relationships and others. A spiritual foundation shifts the focus from 'I' to 'other' as one starts to see life outside of one's self. Beginning to see a HP and its role in life connects one to the reality that there are others out there that break the mind, soul, and spirit free from the trap of Addiction, which says 'It is all about me'.

Spirituality, believing in a force other than oneself, and connecting with this, brings with it feelings of hope, faith, gratitude, and serenity. Hope is the feeling that what is wanted can be had or that events will turn out for the best. Hope is different than expectation, where we are looking for a particular outcome. Hope is trusting that your HP and recovery will move things forward in the way that they need to, not necessarily always in the way one may want it to. When one is tied to specific expectations about how events, conversations, or relationships will develop, they are already setting themselves up for resentment. Expectations are often called 'premeditated resentments' for this reason.

Faith is part of this process, allowing us to move freely through our lives. It can be overwhelming to trust the universe's plan and relinquish control and expectation. Faith is the antidote to FEAR (False Evidence Appearing Real). Fear is often internally created and is fed by the expectations we have about people, places, and things. Fear can keep us paralyzed and stuck in wondering 'what if'. Hope and faith can break the chains of fear and allow one to live in the moment and accept any possible outcome, recognizing that they are neither 'good' nor 'bad', but what needs to be at that moment. Ability to do this can often lead to a sense of gratitude. Even when outcomes are uncomfortable and it may be difficult to see the Higher Power plan in them, one can be thankful and ready to show appreciation for the guidance. With hope, faith, and gratitude comes a sense of serenity; a beautiful feeling of tranquility in which the mind, body, and soul are quiet and calm. The mind is not racing with 'what ifs' and trying to control or predict outcomes. Rather, it is taking in the information being provided and letting it go.

Gratitude: The quality of being thankful; readiness to show appreciation for and to return kindness.

How can you practice gratitude on an ongoing basis?

_____

_____

_____

_____

_____

Faith: Complete trust in someone or something.

How can you practice faithfulness on an ongoing basis?

_____

_____

_____

_____

_____

Serenity: The state of being calm, peaceful and tranquil.

How can you practice serenity on an ongoing basis?

_____

_____

_____

_____

_____

Within Addiction, spirituality is commonly the most underdeveloped aspect of self and the first to take a backseat when relapse vulnerability builds. Meditation, prayer, journaling, and reflection begin to wane as the disease waxes. This is more reason for spirituality to be a focal point in recovery, as it provides valuable information as to the state of the disease. If spirituality is strong, disease vulnerability is lowered. If spirituality is shaky, disease vulnerability is higher.

Spiritual recommendations

- Connection with spirituality through individual reflection, prayer

- Reflecting on daily "coincidences" to identify Higher Power role in daily living

- Attending or creating spiritual ceremonies, group gatherings

- Reading and exploration

- Writing and tracking spiritual beliefs, as well as challenges coming up

- Talking about spiritual journey with recovery supports, spiritual mentor (if available)

- Meditation to connect with universal consciousness

- Spending time in nature, appreciating the beauty around you

- (Re)connecting with the universe and the idea that you are supported and not alone. This is often lost or drastically impacted during active Addiction and relapse

What values are compromised when the disease is active?

_____

_____

_____

_____

_____

How do you maintain awareness of and commitment to your values?

_____

_____

_____

_____

_____

How do you maintain connection with people, places and things that provide meaning in your life?

_____

_____

_____

_____

_____

What examples or evidence are you aware of in yourself and others that recovery is possible?

_____

_____

_____

_____

_____

List recovery actions that you would now have more confidence in taking.

Biologically:

_____

_____

_____

_____
_____

Psychologically:

_____
_____
_____
_____
_____

Socially:

_____
_____
_____
_____
_____

Spiritually:

_____
_____
_____
_____
_____

What does powerlessness mean to you?

_____
_____
_____
_____
_____

What does empowerment mean to you?

_____
_____
_____
_____
_____

Realistic recovery involves

- *Challenges and bumps in the road*

- *"Progress, not perfection"*

- *Daily work on self (journaling, meditating, reflecting, being challenged by others, going to meetings, praying)*

- *Dealing with emotions, money, relationships, work, and life differently*

- *Changes to lifestyle over time*

Typically, in the early days of recovery (first three months or 90 days), the focus often tends to be living and breathing recovery. People are focusing on abstinence and engaging in a new healthy lifestyle. This is a time when lots of emotions are present, which can feel overwhelming and daunting. Some people experience the 'pink cloud' when life immediately feels so much better but many people do not.

From 3–12 months, recovery routine starts to feel more natural and comfortable. New connections are forming; people are starting to explore other activities and recovery options. Cravings may be less; spirituality and relationship questions come to the forefront. Exploring feelings of shame and fear become more prevalent as the focus isn't just on abstinence anymore.

Recovery beyond the first year looks different for everyone. Cravings may resurface. Issues with food, sex, love, relationships may become more prominent. Now there is an engrained recovery routine, but complacency can easily kick in. Overall, there is more stability in self, relationships, emotions, and thinking.

Where are you currently at in your recovery journey?

_____

_____

_____

_____

_____

If you are progressing in sobriety but not noticing these changes happening, you may need to re-evaluate your recovery plan and make adjustments as needed. Often difficulties with emotions and relationships can contribute to feeling 'stuck'.

Powerlessness. When the 12-Step programs were developed, the founders intuitively and practically understood that surrendering to the disease of Addiction and acknowledging both *powerlessness* and *unmanageability* were the necessary first steps to getting well. Hence, step one states, "We admitted that we were powerless over [our Addiction] and that our lives had become unmanageable." What makes the process of surrender so important? The disease of Addiction is all about control. The disease feeds the mind information that 'If I try harder, do better, am more motivated, things will be okay.' This is the starting point of shame because, of course, the disease is uncontrollable and unpredictable once it has been activated. Only when the illusion of control has been let go of can the process of recovery unfold. It is important that one understand the disease as well as engage in recovery, but even still there were still be symptoms of the disease that cannot be controlled. For example, after being in recovery for 10 years from substances, Clark noticed that he was continuing to use pornography and masturbation as an escape from stress, shame, and relationship turmoil in his life. He began to pursue abstinence from these sexual behaviours and, from time to come, noticed cravings to act out would come. Clark realized he cannot control these cravings or make them go away. Instead, he has to accept and acknowledge them and continue to work in his recovery.

What are your ongoing symptoms of active Addiction?

_____

_____

_____

_____

_____

How accepting of these symptoms you? Which ones are you fighting against and hoping will disappear?

_____

_____

_____

_____

_____

Although it may seem counterintuitive, empowerment, which is having the courage and confidence to change the things you can, only happens when one accepts powerlessness over people, places and things that one cannot change.

List people that are important to you that you would like to change but cannot:

_____

_____

_____

_____

_____

List places that you still want to go to but are now aware that are detrimental to your recovery:

_____

_____

_____

_____

_____

List things (activities) that compromise your recovery:

_____

_____

_____

_____

_____

Abstinence beyond substances

Abstinence is the ongoing pursuit of restraint from all mood-altering substances (no use) and behaviours (boundaries). In recovery, it is important to not be using any substances that interfere with Addiction (e.g., illicit drugs, tobacco, alcohol, certain prescription or over-the-counter medications) so if you are unsure, it is recommended you discuss this further with your primary physician.

When exploring abstinence beyond substances, this can become much more challenging for people as abstinence is different for everyone. The three circles is a very beneficial tool for people to use in recovery and can be used with sex, relationships, food, work, physical activity, spending, etc., i.e., problematic behaviours.

Green Zone: people, places and things (activities) that support health and recovery.

Grey Zone: is the area you are unsure about; this is the zone you haven't figured out yet so it will be important to explore further. It will be important to continually ask yourself. Do these people, places, things (activities) support my recovery or feed my disease?

Red Zone: is the abstinence zone. These are clearly defined people, places and things (activities) that you know activate your disease; they are the ones that trigger obsession, rumination, the desire for 'more'.

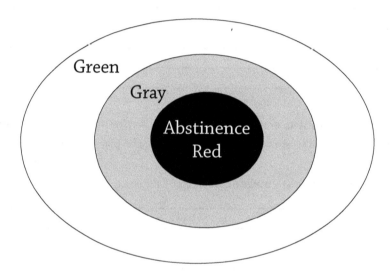

Who are people, places and things/activities that belong in your red zone?

_____

_____

_____

_____

_____

Who are people, places and things/activities currently in your grey zone?

_____

_____

_____

_____

_____

Who are people, places and things/activities in your green zone that support your recovery?

_____

_____

_____

_____
_____

BEING AND DOING (IN RECOVERY)

As discussed, activities in holistic recovery include taking care of the body – exercise, healthy eating, getting adequate sleep, attending to any physical health problems; and the mind and spirit – meditation, journaling, cultivate awareness of addictive thinking, sitting with feelings, praying, admitting powerlessness and practising letting go. Other activities such as pursuing hobbies, community support meetings, reaching out to others, putting up boundaries in relationships, disconnecting from unhealthy people, trying new activities, being assertive, working the twelve steps, and developing new sober relationships are all possibilities within the holistic recovery framework. This is just a sample of all the recovery actions available and they all require commitment and practice. Not all of these will work for everyone, but developing a toolbox in recovery is important. Gone are the days of relying on one go-to escape, reward, or relief mechanism, which is what Addiction is all about. What will work for self-care and nurturing today in recovery may not help as much tomorrow, but that does not mean it is not a helpful tool to keep in the toolbox. Thankfully, there are other tools that can be tried out when the hammer is not enough.

"Developing a toolbox in recovery is important."

What does doing versus being in recovery mean to you?

_____
_____
_____
_____
_____

In early recovery, it is not uncommon for people to 'do recovery' meaning they take action and focus on the doing part, checking off their 'to do list' to get them accomplished (e.g., 90 meetings in 90 days). Over time, it's important that there's a shift to 'being in recovery', which is when people start to feel connected to themselves, others and their life in recovery. There is a sense of belonging. If this shift does not occur, it will continue to feel like a chore rather than a change in lifestyle that is sustainable.

Are you being or doing recovery currently?

_____
_____
_____
_____
_____

RECOVERY PLAN

It is essential to have a recovery plan to guide your daily activities rather than trying to do things on the fly. To help you build your own personal recovery plan, review the following list and check off the activities you are already doing or aspire to do:

- ☐ Drink 1L+ of water/day
- ☐ Eat nutritiously
- ☐ Meditate
- ☐ Journal
- ☐ Draw, paint, create
- ☐ Song or poetry writing
- ☐ Assertiveness
- ☐ Hobbies (sports, crafts, music, book club, other: _____)
- ☐ 12-Step meetings
- ☐ Other community meetings (e.g., SMART, Refuge)
- ☐ Say no
- ☐ Let go
- ☐ Prayer

- ☐ Disconnect from unhealthy people
- ☐ Set boundaries
- ☐ Identify my needs
- ☐ Exercise 3–5 times/week
- ☐ Equine therapy
- ☐ Reach out to friends, family and healthy supports
- ☐ Individual therapy
- ☐ Group therapy
- ☐ Feel the feelings
- ☐ Mindfulness
- ☐ Deep breathing
- ☐ Abstinence from mood altering substances

- ☐ Admitting powerlessness
- ☐ Learn more about Addiction
- ☐ Meet with clergy/spiritual leaders
- ☐ Hypnotherapy
- ☐ Acupuncture, other complementary treatments
- ☐ Retreats, activity groups
- ☐ Accept
- ☐ Go to church
- ☐ Yoga
- ☐ Have fun!

Now that you have an idea of the activities you are doing, as well as would like to do, you can look at building your personalized recovery plan and schedule. Below we have included a sample recovery schedule for people currently working, as well as for people who are not currently working, whether that be because you are retired, unemployed, a stay at home caregiver, or on medical leave. Keep in mind that not all of these activities will fit for you, nor do they need to be done at the times recommended. This is a sample and is designed to give you some ideas and structure of things you could do for your own recovery. If you feel overwhelmed looking at the schedules, pick out two key activities each day that would be most meaningful and start by putting those into your own routine, then build from there. Have a read through the sample schedules and then use the blank template to create your own.

Sample schedule for someone working:

Time	Monday	Tuesday	Wednesday	Thursday	Friday	Saturday	Sunday
6:30-8:30am	Wake-up, meditate, morning reading, shower and hygiene, eat breakfast	Wake-up, meditate, morning reading, shower and hygiene, eat breakfast, attend early morning 12-Step meeting	Wake-up, meditate, morning reading, shower and hygiene, eat breakfast	Wake-up, meditate, morning reading, shower and hygiene, eat breakfast	Wake-up, meditate, morning reading, shower and hygiene, eat breakfast	Wake-up, meditate, morning reading, shower and hygiene, eat breakfast	Wake-up, meditate, morning reading, get ready, eat breakfast
8:30-12:00pm	Work	Work	Work	Work	Work, attend individual therapy appointment	Walk, go to a 12-step meeting	Go to church
12:00-1:00pm	Lunch, walk outside	Lunch, yoga class	Lunch, 12-Step meeting	Lunch, go for a walk	Lunch	Lunch out after meeting	Lunch at home
1:00-5:00pm	Work, break for snack, walk around mid-afternoon, reach out to recovery buddy	Work, break for snack, walk around mid-afternoon, feelings check-in ("how am I feeling today?")	Work, break for snack, walk around mid-afternoon, feelings check-in	Work, break for snack, walk around mid-afternoon	Work, break for snack, walk around mid-afternoon, feelings check-in	Fun! (Art class, physical activity, movie, etc.)	Relax at home, clean, read, cook
5:00-6:00pm	Come home, meditate, prepare and eat dinner	Come home, meditate, prepare and eat dinner	Come home, meditate, prepare and eat dinner	Come home, meditate, prepare and eat dinner	Come home, meditate, prepare and eat dinner	Prepare and eat dinner	Cook dinner for guests
6:00-7:00pm	Relax, read/watch TV, prepare lunch for tomorrow	Relax, read/watch TV, prepare lunch for tomorrow	Relax, read/watch TV, prepare lunch for tomorrow	Relax, read/watch TV, prepare lunch for tomorrow	Relax, read/watch TV	Relax at home or go out with people who are healthy for me	Relax, read/watch TV, prepare lunch for tomorrow
7:00-9:00pm	Go to 12-step meeting	Stay home, relax, do stretching	Go to the gym, relax	Group therapy	Go to 12-step meeting	Keep enjoying my evening	Attend 12-Step meeting
9:00-10:00pm	Bedtime ritual: journal feelings, read, pray	Bedtime ritual: journal feelings, read, pray	Bedtime ritual: journal feelings, read, pray	Bedtime ritual: journal feelings, read, pray	Bedtime ritual: journal feelings, read, pray	Bedtime ritual: journal feelings, read, pray	Bedtime ritual: journal feelings, read, pray
10:00pm	Bedtime	Bedtime	Bedtime	Bedtime	Bedtime	Bedtime	Bedtime

Sample schedule when work is not involved:

Time	Monday	Tuesday	Wednesday	Thursday	Friday	Saturday	Sunday
6:30–8:30 a.m.	Wake-up, meditate, morning reading, shower and hygiene, eat breakfast	Wake-up, meditate, morning readings, shower and hygiene, eat breakfast	Wake-up, meditate, morning reading, shower and hygiene, eat breakfast	Wake-up, meditate, morning reading, shower and hygiene, eat breakfast	Wake-up, meditate, morning reading, shower and hygiene, eat breakfast	Wake-up, meditate, morning reading, shower and hygiene, eat breakfast	Wake-up, meditate, morning reading, shower and hygiene, eat breakfast
8:30–12:00 p.m.	Go to the gym and a 12-Step meeting	Errands, medical appointment	Go to the gym and a 12-Step meeting	Yoga class, errands	Go to the gym and a 12-Step meeting	Activity class (art, cooking, hiking, etc.)	Read, walk, spend quiet time with self
12:00–1:00 p.m.	Lunch, walk outside	Lunch	Lunch with a recovery buddy	Lunch, go for a walk	Lunch	Lunch	Lunch
1:00–5:00 p.m.	Attend to house chores, organization. Meditate	Phone contact with recovery buddy, reading. Meditate	Errands, appointments, relaxation. Meditate	Go to a 12-Step meeting. Meditate	Self-care (fun activity, gentle exercise, etc.) Meditate	Time with family and friends. Meditate	Relax at home, clean, read, garden, art. Meditate
5:00–6:00 p.m.	Prepare and eat dinner	Prepare and eat dinner	Come home, prepare and eat dinner	Come home, prepare and eat dinner	Come home, prepare and eat dinner	Come home, prepare and eat dinner	Prepare and eat dinner
6:00–7:00 p.m.	Relax, read/ watch TV/ puzzle/ game	Relax, read/ watch TV/ puzzle/ game	Relax, read/ watch TV/ puzzle/ game	Relax, read/ watch TV/ puzzle game	Relax, read/ watch TV/ puzzle/ game	Outing with friends or family	Relax, read/ watch TV/ puzzle/board game
7:00–9:00 p.m.	Stay home, relax, do life tasks (taxes, bills, etc.)	Go to 12-Step meeting	Enjoy a leisurely walk outside, read	Group therapy	Hobby time (crafts, music, sports)	Keep enjoying my evening	Keep enjoying my evening, converse with others
9:00–10:00 p.m.	Bedtime ritual: journal feelings, read, pray	Bedtime ritual: journal feelings, read, pray	Bedtime ritual: journal feelings, read, pray	Bedtime ritual: journal feelings, read, pray	Bedtime ritual: journal feelings, read, pray	Bedtime ritual: journal feelings, read, pray	Bedtime ritual: journal feelings, read, pray
10:00 p.m.	Bedtime	Bedtime	Bedtime	Bedtime	Bedtime	Bedtime	Bedtime

Blank recovery schedule template to fill in:

Time	Monday	Tuesday	Wednesday	Thursday	Friday	Saturday	Sunday
6:30–8:30 a.m.							
8:30–12:00 p.m.							
12:00–1:00 p.m.							
1:00–5:00 p.m.							
5:00–6:00 p.m.							
6:00–7:00 p.m.							
7:00–9:00 p.m.							
9:00–10:00 p.m.							
10:00 p.m.							

In this schedule you are able to fill in your activities and the "anchors" for your recovery. Meaning, the key activities that keep you grounded at this point in time and that are essentials for health. It is also important to put these into your day timer, phone calendar or wherever you organize yourself so that you are reminded and visually aware of your recovery priorities.

GOAL SETTING

In active Addiction, goals and priorities become skewed to substance and problem behaviour pursuit and use. A helpful tool for goal setting is SMART. This technique was originally printed in a management magazine and created by George Doran, Arthur Miller, and James Cunningham. It can easily be extrapolated from a workplace context into a recovery one and is a helpful way to approach goal setting.

S=SPECIFIC
M=MEASURABLE
A=ATTAINABLE
R=RELEVANT
T=TIME-BOUND

Let us walk through the example of healthy eating using SMART goals.

Example Goal: I want to eat healthier

Specific (can you define the goal as much as possible so it is not vague and arbitrary?): I am going to consume two litres of unsweetened water per day as well as eat three meals and two snacks

Measurable (can you attach a tangible component to the goal in order to be able to track progress?): I can track how many meals and snacks I am eating per day as well as how much water I am drinking

Attainable (can you evaluate the realism of the goal?): I believe these goals are attainable and realistic for me right now as I have already started to focus on water consumption and improvement of eating habits in the past few months, but so far it has been vague and undefined

Relevant (does this goal fit within your current recovery plan and lifestyle?): I am aware of the physical damage my substance use took on my body and am hoping to improve strength and energy. This is a helpful goal in addition to the recovery work I have already been doing for the past eight months. I have also discussed this with my sponsor and medical doctor

Time-bound (what timeframe are you looking at this goal over?): I will track my progress for one month and re-evaluate at that time what is working and where the challenges are.

Now come up with two of your own goals and write them out using the SMART format

1. Goal:

   Specific:

   Measurable:

   Attainable:

   Relevant:

   Time-bound:

2. Goal:

   Specific:

   Measurable:

   Attainable:

   Relevant:

Time-bound:

There are many challenges that come in goal-setting when Addiction is involved, including issues with motivation, consistency, unrealistic standards, shame, and the pursuit of instant gratification. It is important to use your support network to process the challenges that come up along the way as well as seek feedback, recognizing that at times your brain may be lying or feeding you misinformation. For example, it may tell you that your eating is healthy but when you look at all your snacks that are filled with sugar, others may be able to see something that you are missing that could be aggravating your disease and not serving your recovery.

The process of recovery can only begin once the first step has been taken by the person struggling with Addiction, and that is the step of willingness.

On a scale of 1–10 (not willing-very willing), where is your current willingness to take action on the two SMART goals you outlined before?

WILLINGNESS

All of the recovery actions discussed above are well intentioned and can produce phenomenal results, but only once willingness to change has been reached. For some, this willingness comes when they hit rock-bottom, meaning the lowest point in one's Addiction where there has usually been a significant event that speaks to the progression of Addiction in life. Job loss, marital breakdown, children being apprehended by child services, near-death experiences, bankruptcy, and homelessness are all stark examples of the depths this disease can take one to. Not everyone reaches a bottom like this before entering recovery, and not everyone who reaches this kind of bottom proceeds to develop the willingness to get well.

What does willingness look like for you?

_____

_____

_____

_____

_____

Are you willing to take action and make the changes in your life to become healthier?

_____

_____

_____

_____

_____

What are the barriers to your willingness to engage in recovery?

_____

_____

_____

_____

_____

Willingness or readiness to take action is an individual process and looks different for everyone. Whenever and wherever the willingness begins is also where the shift begins from active disease to recovery.

Key messages

- Recovery is best achieved through a combination of self-management, mutual support, and professional care provided by trained and certified professionals.

- Considering Addiction as a bio-psycho-social-spiritual disease is also a useful approach for recovery.

- A bio-psycho-social-spiritual framework of holistic recovery optimizes outcomes.

- It is essential to have a recovery plan to proactively guide daily activities rather than trying to do things on the fly.

- Part of the recovery plan is to set realistic, healthy goals as a necessary part of the lifestyle shift. This whole process of recovery can only begin once the first step has been taken and that is the step of willingness.

Action steps for Chapter 6 (follow through after chapter exercises)

In this chapter you have learned that recovery plans are tailored to the individual and do not come in pre-determined packages. We would encourage you to revisit your recovery plan and activities regularly (at a minimum every three months) to re-evaluate how you are feeling, what you are doing for recovery, and your ability to be comfortable in yourself. It would be important to re-evaluate this yourself as well as talk about it with one or more of your recovery supports to also get feedback about the changes others are noticing and where there may be some stagnancy happening.

Chapter 7: RAiAR as a Platform for Recovery

"Faith is taking the first step even when you don't see the whole staircase."
—Rev. Dr. Martin Luther King Jr.

Remember Addiction is Addiction Responsible Recovery (RAiAR)

RAiAR is a mutual support program which offers weekly, closed, small group (maximum of 9 participants) meetings, with occasional speaker meetings, to assist people in recovery from Addiction. There are two moderators at each group meeting to encourage sharing, promote constructive feedback and guide the discussion to assist in recovery growth. RAiAR is a complement to 12-Step programs and people will be able to appreciate how the recovery concepts can be reinforced utilizing a variety of approaches.

The first three steps of RAiAR focus on willingness and awareness of the disease of Addiction. They are:

1. I am willing to consider that Addiction is a primary, chronic disease that is progressive, relapsing and often causes disability and premature death.

2. I am willing to consider that Addiction manifests in biological, psychological, social, and spiritual dimensions with the use of substances and/or addictive behaviours.

3. I am willing to consider that recovery is possible through support from other people and connection to a Higher Power.

What doubts do you have about the primary, chronic nature of Addiction?

_____
_____
_____
_____
_____
_____
_____

What evidence do you have from your own life or of your loved one that indicates that the disease of Addiction is progressive and relapsing?

_____
_____
_____
_____
_____

_____

_____

What doubts do you have about support from others and/or a Higher Power?

_____

_____

_____

_____

_____

_____

_____

List the specific harms to yourself you have become aware of:

Biologically:

_____

_____

_____

Psychologically:

_____

_____

_____

Socially:

_____

_____

_____

Spiritually:

_____

_____

_____

The middle three steps of RAiAR focus on action once willingness has been clarified and established as a foundation. These are:

4. *I can and will cultivate awareness of the harm caused by my disease of addiction in my life to me and others.*

5. *I can and will cultivate awareness of my connection to others and my Higher Power through honest sharing.*

6. *I can and will actively share, from a strictly personal perspective, to surrender shame, let go of control and accept life on life's terms.*

Harms related to Addiction occur along biological, psychological, social, and spiritual dimensions and healing in recovery requires ever growing awareness and steady, consistent action.

Make a list of people in your life that harms may have happened to due to your disease along the four dimensions listed above.

Harms to me and others:

Biologically:

_____
_____
_____

Psychologically:

_____
_____
_____

Socially:

_____
_____
_____

Spiritually:

_____
_____
_____

If the relationship is in the past, it will require talking to a trusted recovering peer to help you in becoming more aware. If the relationship is ongoing and there is trust there, an open-ended exploration to listen to your loved one's perspective will help you expand your awareness. It is essential that blaming and shaming does not happen during this process. If any blame or shame arises, a step back with appropriate boundaries would be essential to prevent further harm. It is critical for both parties engaging in this kind of exploration that the aim is better understanding rather than apologizing, seeking or granting 'forgiveness'.

What is my awareness of connection to others and/or my Higher Power?

_____
_____
_____
_____
_____

What are my barriers to sharing honestly, surrendering control, and dealing with shame?

_____
_____
_____

_____

_____

As much as honesty, open-mindedness, and willingness bring awareness, action is needed to bring more awareness, as is taking responsibility, which is part of the last three steps of RAiAR.

The last three steps of RAiAR focus on clarifying one's responsibility in recovery. They are:

7. *I am responsible for being honest and practicing humility to the best of my ability.*

8. *I am responsible for boundaries and balance in my life.*

9. *I am responsible for recovery action and staying in process, the outcomes will be determined by the grace of my Higher Power.*

List examples of honesty and humility that are part of your daily practice now:

_____

_____

_____

_____

_____

List examples of boundaries with people, places and things in your life now:

_____

_____

_____

_____

_____

_____

List examples of biological, psychological, social, and spiritual balance in your life now:

_____

_____

_____

_____

_____

_____

List examples of your connection to your Higher Power now:

_____

_____

_____
_____
_____
_____
_____

List examples of outcomes in your life that you see represent the grace of your Higher Power:

_____
_____
_____
_____
_____
_____
_____

The Higher Power connection is ever present in everyone's life, as it is the life force (laws of nature) without which our existence is not possible. When one says that they are not spiritual or do not believe in a Higher Power, it actually means that they are unaware of and/or are taking their existence for granted. Over-intellectualization and false belief that 'I am in control of my thinking, behaviour, and destiny' is actually an example of addictive thinking that is ever present in someone who is lacking in humility and caught up in grandiosity. It is essential to appreciate that awareness of the Higher Power connection comes from the inside of each of us and has to be cultivated personally rather than being imposed externally. Religions around the world have tried to impose 'social-spiritual sanctions' to keep people in line with fear and shame. This approach can bring short-term results on the surface but invariably leads to long-term resentments and anger that eventually leads to reform individually and collectively.

What examples can you think of in your experience where God or Higher Power concepts were externally imposed on you?

_____
_____
_____
_____

How did you feel about the external impositions?

_____
_____
_____
_____

What did you do or are you doing with those feelings?

_____
_____
_____
_____
_____

Appendix A provides additional information about the structure, format and background information to RAiAR if you are interested in learning more for yourself as a potential participant or as someone keen to start a similar group in your area.

Key messages

- RAiAR is a mutual support program to assist people in recovery from Addiction.

- RAiAR is a complement to 12-Step programs.

- There are nine steps, the first three steps focus on willingness and awareness of the disease of Addiction.

- The middle three steps focus on action once willingness has been clarified and established as a foundation.

- The last three steps focus on clarifying one's responsibility in recovery.

Action steps for Chapter 7 (follow through after chapter exercises)

In this chapter you have been exposed to another mutual support program called RAiAR. Whether you are a member of a 12-Step fellowship or not, we would encourage you to keep exploring all of the group and mutual support options available in your city and surrounding area and participate as possible to get a flavour for the differences as well as what can work for you. As you move forward in your recovery, you may feel so inclined to start your own group, whether a 12-Step fellowship meeting, RAiAR group or other mutual support program.

Chapter 8: Family Matters

"Family isn't about whose blood you carry,
it's who you love and who loves you back."
—*Unknown*

Whether you are a person with Addiction or a family member of someone who has Addiction, this entire workbook will have benefit for you. In particular, this chapter allows you to explore your family relationships in more depth. You will be able to see your part in interactions as well as how to cultivate healthier dynamics with people in your family through boundaries, healthy communication, and interdependence.

FAMILY ROLES

There are common roles that people in families living with Addiction take on that become adaptive, a way to survive, but that may impact quality of life and relationship. Here we will explore these roles and how to move out of them to healthier ones. Complete the self-test below to see what role(s) best fit for you:

Roles in the Family Self-test:

Check all the statements that apply to you in each section.
Section 1

- ☐ *I have or have had issues with out of control use of drugs, alcohol, or problem behaviours such as sex, food, exercise, spending, relationships, etc.*
- ☐ *I have a lot of pain and shame for the things I have done in my life*
- ☐ *I feel inadequate the majority of the time*
- ☐ *I have been diagnosed with Addiction/substance dependence or acknowledge having this*

- ☐ *I find it hard to deal with and express my feelings in a healthy and appropriate way*
- ☐ *I am a perfectionist*
- ☐ *I isolate, particularly in difficult times*
- ☐ *I struggle with stress and how to cope with it*
- ☐ *I think I am great, healthy, and no changes need to be made in my life*

Section 2

- ☐ *I find it difficult to see people I love suffering*
- ☐ *I feel it is my responsibility to help people around me, no matter what*
- ☐ *I find myself lying to others about what is really happening in my family, at home, and with me*
- ☐ *I want the outside world to think everything is okay, even if it is not*

- ☐ *I have sometimes turned a blind eye to my loved one's acting out with substances or problem behaviours*
- ☐ *I am aware my loved one has an issue with Addiction but I have continued to drink, use drugs, and/or engage in their problem behaviour with them*

☐ *I have seen behaviours in my loved one that are worrisome to me, but I have not said anything to them about it*

☐ *I have made excuses for my loved one before with social engagements, family functions, work, or other appointments when they have been unable to attend*

☐ *I have monitored the amount my loved one was drinking, using, or their problem behaviour*

☐ *I have tried to control or stop my loved one's engagement with their problem behaviour or substance*

☐ *I do not have time for myself because I am so busy looking after others*

Section 3

☐ *I strive for high achievement and excellent performance*

☐ *I go out of my way to be the best*

☐ *I am an incredibly successful individual*

☐ *I highly value my accomplishments as they will make others happy with me and my family*

☐ *I use my own accomplishments to hide the issues in my family and/or self*

☐ *I feel responsible for fixing my family's pain*

☐ *I overwork or would describe myself as a work-a-holic*

☐ *I feel inadequate unless I succeed*

☐ *I get self-worth from being special and successful*

☐ *No amount of achievement is ever enough; I am always striving for more*

☐ *I have distanced myself from my family because I am ashamed and/or feel different than them*

Section 4

☐ *I value breaking the rules and going against the grain*

☐ *I have often been blamed or taken punishment for something that was not my fault*

☐ *I would rather be punished than see my family members blamed*

☐ *I feel a lot of hurt and guilt*

☐ *My family blames me for the problems happening within the family*

☐ *I have issues with people in authority*

☐ *I have encountered problems with teachers, principals, parents, and/or the law*

☐ *I have felt suicidal or attempted suicide*

☐ *I am defiant towards others*

Section 5

☐ *I use humour to lighten tense or depressed moods*

☐ *I often feel scared in interpersonal situations*

☐ *I am often judged as being immature*

☐ *I have been told that I use humour inappropriately*

☐ *I am popular within my family*

☐ *I enjoy getting attention from others*

☐ *I find pleasure in making people laugh, perhaps have been called the 'class clown'*

☐ *I am quite hyperactive*

☐ *I put myself down to make others feel better*

☐ *I find humour is a great distraction*

☐ *I am there to encourage others and cheer them on*

Section 6

☐ *I am quite withdrawn and described as a 'loner'*

☐ *I am quite distant from my family; they do not pay much attention to me*

☐ *I do not like being in the spotlight or centre of attention*

☐ *I do not feel important or valued by my family*

☐ *I find it difficult to communicate and express myself to others*

☐ *I feel confused and inadequate in relationships*

☐ *I like to be by myself and enjoy activities where I am alone*

☐ *I prefer to be in a fantasy world than the real one*

As you look at your responses, there will likely be one or a few categories where you had more check marks than others. The roles that you had the highest number of check marks for are likely the roles that you have taken on in your family.

Section 1 describes a person with the disease of Addiction. Section 2 is the 'chief enabler or caretaker'. Section 3 is the 'hero'. Section 4 is the 'scapegoat or rebel'. Section 5 is the 'mascot, cheerleader, or clown'. Section 6 is the 'lost child or wallflower' role. Often people have experience in multiple roles, although some are clearly just limited to one role. Neither is better nor worse, right nor wrong. This is intended for cultivating learning and awareness.

Write about your experience in each of the roles you had check marks in.

_____

_____

_____

_____

_____

What did behaviour look like for you when you were active in that role or roles?

_____

_____

_____

_____

_____

What consequences and benefits came with this role or roles?

_____

_____

_____

_____

_____

How did you feel in this role or roles?

_____

_____

_____

_____

_____

Explore your level of satisfaction in this role(s). Do you want to change or stay the same? Explain the motivation behind this.

_____

_____

_____

_____

_____

What would a healthy role in your family look, feel, and sound like?

_____

_____

_____

_____

_____

What steps can you take to move towards this healthy role and away from the dysfunctional one(s)?

_____

_____

_____

_____

_____

To move from unhealthy to healthy roles involves a number of action steps, including boundaries and communication.

BOUNDARIES

Many people, even when recognizing the disease, feel they are responsible for another person's Addiction. They try to control it and hang on to a false belief that they can fix it. This leads to misery and frustration for everyone. This is a false sense of control, for only the individual with Addiction can take accountability and responsibility for their recovery, but it can never be entirely cured or fixed as there will always be symptoms present. Boundaries, knowing where you end and another begins, are key to stepping away from control and embracing recovery.

Below is a boundary quiz. Check any of the statements that are examples of healthy boundaries:

1. *Saying "Stop lying to me"*

2. *Saying "I don't like being lied to. This is the end of our conversation"*

3. *Having an exit strategy if people are drinking or using drugs around you at an event*

4. *Test your recovery strength and stick it out if people are drinking and using drugs around you at an event*

5. *Call and book your loved one into residential treatment as it is obvious they are struggling and so are you as a result of seeing them suffer*

6. *Have a plan for distancing and detaching to keep yourself safe if your loved one's problem behaviour(s) continues*

From the statements above, options number 2, 3 and 6 are the appropriate boundary options. The others involve control and are not set by you, for you, which boundaries always need to be. Boundaries are guidelines, rules, or limits that a person creates to identify what are reasonable, safe, and permissible ways to interact with other people around us and how we will respond when someone pushes those limits. You may notice from the examples that sometimes boundaries can be verbalized (like with option 2) but they do not always have to be (options 3 and 6). Sometimes the verbalization can be part of control, where we are wanting to make sure people understand and are on board with our boundaries rather than just being clear within ourselves that is what we need.

What are my boundaries in relationships with others?

_____

_____

_____

_____
_____
_____
_____

What are my boundaries with myself (and my disease of Addiction)?

_____
_____
_____
_____
_____
_____

What difficulties do I have reinforcing my boundaries?

_____
_____
_____
_____
_____
_____

People typically have internal and external boundaries and there is no obligation to share any of these with others. For example, an internal boundary is "not engaging in thoughts of my ex-girlfriend." An external boundary is "not engaging with her such as texting or commenting on her social media posts." Both boundaries are set by you, for you. We often hear people tell us that someone in their life didn't respect their boundary. As mentioned previously, this just provides information on where the other person is at and the intention of boundaries is to keep yourself safe/healthy rather than change others actions or behaviours towards you.

It is often easier to make other people happy and focus on what they want and need rather than doing this for us. Boundaries are all about knowing what is important and necessary to us and honouring that within ourselves, whether we verbally express it to someone else or not. We do not have to verbally express our boundary; actions speak much louder than words.

Think of a specific boundary you have set or would like to set. Write it down.

_____
_____
_____
_____

How can you reinforce this boundary through action rather than words?

_____
_____
_____

_____

_____

Boundaries:

- *Are essential in all relationships*

- *Different than expectations*

- ***Expectations****: when we expect somebody else to act differently*

- ***Boundaries****: when we act differently as a result of an internal line we have set, what you will/will not accept for yourself*

In terms of supporting others, boundaries are crucial to be able to move from sympathetic caretaker (dysfunctional role) to empathetic helper (functional role). For example, a sympathetic caretaker may be trying to control the other person's behaviour or inadvertently enabling them in their disease rather than looking at how they can realistically provide support and what their limits are.

Do you currently have a person in your life who is struggling somehow? Write about them here.

_____

_____

_____

_____

_____

_____

_____

What are you able to offer to that person for support?

_____

_____

_____

_____

What are you unable/unwilling to do for them?

_____

_____

_____

_____

Boundaries require an appreciation that another person cannot do for someone what (s)he needs to do for themselves. Recovery is a key example of that. If a person does not want to engage in health and recovery, they will not. To develop and enforce boundaries, clarity around the question of 'who am I?' and healthy communication are essential.

EMOTIONAL HEALING

The healing process for family members is just as important as for those with the disease of Addiction. There are many feelings generated for family members of people with Addiction, which include fear, resentment, anger, guilt, and shame. It is important to be mindful of all feelings that come up and to not judge them or label them as 'good' or 'bad.' Feelings provide us with valuable information that is necessary to listen to in order to heal emotionally and be on the path to health. If you are a family member doing this workbook, it would also be important for you to complete the activities in the 'Addictive Feeling' chapter that deals extensively with each of the feelings below.

Fear. Untreated Addiction is especially scary to the outside observer as you see a loved one who is out of control, unreasonable, and so completely different than who you know your loved one to be. Even as your loved one finds treatment and recovery, the fear may continue or have long-term consequences.

Write down all of the fears you have/have had regarding your loved one(s) with Addiction (or self):

_____

_____

_____

_____

_____

Write down all of your other life fears (relationships, finances, job security, health, etc.):

_____

_____

_____

_____

_____

How have you coped with these fears?

_____

_____

_____

_____

_____

_____

Look at each of your coping mechanisms and put whether it has been Healthy (H), Unhealthy (U) or Both (B) beside each one.

For the unhealthy (U) or both (B) coping mechanisms, what can you do differently to make coping healthier for you?

_____

_____

_____

_____

_____

_____

It is important to explore your fears and sit with them, rather than run away from them or convince yourself that they are gone because you or your loved one is getting better. The same is true for resentments you may be carrying.

Resentment. For family members who do not have the disease of Addiction, it is difficult to understand what their loved one is going through. They see the carnage of Addiction: the lies, deceit, 'failures', broken promises, and destruction which can all lead to resentment building up over time. For the person with the disease, they are often resentful towards themselves (mistaking their disease and self as the same) as well as others for their pushiness, judgement, control, and lack of support.

How has your or your family member(s) Addiction impacted you?

_____
_____
_____
_____
_____

How did you see your or your family member(s) Addiction impacting the family?

_____
_____
_____
_____
_____

How did you feel about witnessing Addiction in your family?

_____
_____
_____
_____
_____

If you did not have obvious Addiction in your family as you were growing up, what was happening (or not happening) that generated resentments for you? (E.g., neglect, abuse, pressure to perform, lack of emotional availability, enmeshment).

_____
_____
_____
_____
_____

Make a list of all of the resentments you are carrying towards your family member(s) who have Addiction:

_____
_____

_____

_____

_____

Make a list of all of the resentments you are carrying towards your closest family members (even those who do not seem to have Addiction):

_____

_____

_____

_____

_____

Make a list of all the resentments you are carrying towards yourself (and your disease of Addiction, if applicable):

_____

_____

_____

_____

_____

How have you coped with these resentments over time?

_____

_____

_____

_____

_____

What behaviours and other feelings has your resentment led you to? (E.g., anger outbursts, self-harm, avoidance, control, manipulation).

_____

_____

_____

_____

_____

Are you willing to start trying to let go of the resentments you are carrying towards your family?

_____

_____

_____

_____

_____

What are the obstacles to your willingness?

_____

_____

_____

_____

_____

If you are willing, how can you start to let go of the resentments you are carrying towards your family? Yourself?

_____

_____

_____

_____

_____

If you are not willing, what harm do you think hanging on to your resentment may have on you and your relationships?

_____

_____

_____

_____

_____

What are you getting out of hanging on to your resentment?

_____

_____

_____

_____

_____

As with other emotions, like fear, anger, and shame, hanging on to resentment causes the most damage to the person who has them. While it may be strangely comforting and familiar to hang on to these emotions because they have been around for so long, for short-and long-term health it is important to look at letting go, which is of course easier said than done but very rewarding when it happens. As the saying goes, "hanging onto anger is like drinking poison and expecting the other person to die."

"We need to carry hope for the future but hope is flexible and adaptive to the process, whereas expectations are rigid and defined."

Letting go of expectations. This is the key to letting go of resentments. If we carry within us the expectation of an outcome (e.g., that abstinence will equal health and happiness or that the person with Addiction is fully to blame for the relationship issues so them getting better means no more issues), then we are setting ourselves up for disappointment and more resentment.

What expectations are you carrying for your own life? (Note, often expectations have the word 'should' in them).

_____

_____

_____

_____

What expectations are you carrying for your loved one(s) with Addiction's life, health, and recovery?

_____

_____

_____

_____

_____

How have these expectations benefitted you?

_____

_____

_____

_____

_____

How have these expectations harmed you?

_____

_____

_____

_____

_____

How do you feel when your expectations are not met?

_____

_____

_____

_____

_____

How is hope different from expectation for you?

_____

_____

_____

_____

_____

How can you move into hope and away from expectation?

_____

_____

_____

_____

_____

Letting go of expectations means trusting that you will get what you need, which is not always what we thought we needed (or wanted).

Anger. When we are carrying resentments, which come from expectations, we are also carrying anger. Anger can be directed inwards, outwards, or both.

When I am angry, what do I do - act out? suppress feelings? or both?

_____
_____
_____
_____
_____

How often are you angry? How come?

_____
_____
_____
_____

As discussed in previous chapters, anger is a composite emotion comprised of many feelings that come together as anger.

When you are angry, you are also feeling …

_____
_____
_____
_____

How can you cope with your anger more constructively?

_____
_____
_____
_____

Often, anger is made worse by feelings of guilt and shame that we are carrying that we project onto the people around us. Therefore, it is also important to explore what these feelings look and feel like for you and how to cope with them in a healthy way.

Guilt and Shame. As discussed in the Addictive Feeling chapter, it is important to distinguish between guilt and shame because people often confuse the two when, in fact, they are very different experiences. Guilt is a thinking process about action: 'I did bad.' Whereas shame says 'I am bad.'

What have you done (or not done) in your life that you feel bad about?

_____

_____

_____

_____

_____

Do these actions make you a flawed, bad, or unlovable person? How?

_____

_____

_____

_____

_____

If you answered 'no' to the last question then you may not be carrying a lot of shame or you have not been able to connect to your shame. It would still be worth doing the questions below regarding shame to see what comes up for you. If you answered 'yes' to the last question, than you are struggling with shame.

Write more about what your shame sounds like. In other words, what is the self-talk in your head on a daily basis?

_____

_____

_____

_____

_____

_____

What does shame feel like in your body?

_____

_____

_____

_____

_____

Draw a picture of what shame looks like to you.

How does shame drive you to act with others?

_____

_____

_____

_____

_____

What more do you believe you should be doing for your loved one?

_____

_____

_____

_____

_____

What does acceptance mean to you?

_____

_____

_____

_____

_____

How can you incorporate acceptance into your behaviours and routine?

_____

_____

_____
_____
_____

Awareness of each of these feelings and how they affect you is an important step in the recovery process. This can be done through talking with peer supports and/or a therapist trained in Addiction in addition to the exploration questions in this workbook. Other helpful activities include journaling, prayer, meditation, reflection, and body scanning to learn more about these feelings.

Reconnecting with or recovering who you are is no easy task and can be facilitated by asking yourself the following questions:

What are my core values? (Examples may include: determination, honesty, integrity, loyalty)

_____
_____
_____
_____
_____

What do I enjoy doing and find fun?

_____
_____
_____
_____
_____

What recharges me? (For instance, does quiet time or doing something with one or two close friends provide you with an influx of energy, or does being engaged in a group activity or lively discussion leave you feeling invigorated?)

_____
_____
_____
_____
_____

What do I feel is my purpose on earth? What would I like to contribute to myself and others?

_____
_____
_____
_____
_____

What do I feel passionate about or have felt passionate about in the past?

_____
_____
_____

_____

_____

What am I looking for in a healthy relationship with myself and others?

_____

_____

_____

_____

_____

You may need to spend time over many months, or longer, talking through and writing out your answers to these questions. The process of disconnecting from yourself took time, so reconnection cannot happen instantly—but will come quicker than you anticipate.

Strengths/affirmations. With an increase in shame and disconnection from self comes a decrease in self-esteem, confidence, and self-worth. Rediscovering and eventually liking and loving yourself are essential for lifelong health and well-being. A simple but powerful way to do this is through affirmations. For best results, it is important to practice affirmations regularly throughout the day because you may have unconsciously developed the habit of negative, destructive self-talk. It will take some time, but is possible, to override this with healthy self-talk. The more conscious time and effort you can put into affirmations and focusing on strength, the more natural this process will become. Examples may include: 'I am strong,' 'I am moving forward at my own pace through change,' or 'I honour who I am and where I am at with love, empathy and compassion.'

To create affirmations, write 'I am' followed by a trait or characteristic you possess. Write down at least 20 of these:

1.

2.

3.

4.

5.

6.

7.

8.

9.

10.

11.

12.

13.

14.

15.

16.

17.

18.

19.

20.

It may take some time for these strengths to become internalized as core truths but our minds are resilient to absorbing this kind of self-talk as an antidote to the destructive self-talk that has occurred for many years. As your sense of self strengthens and recovery progresses, you may notice a shift in your communication, which is essential for healthy relationships.

HEALTHY COMMUNICATION

There are different modes of communication that we must pay attention to when looking at how we interact with others.

Non-verbal communication. Our body language and listening skills are key in the messages we convey during interactions with others. For healthy communication, it is important to convey that we are open, engaged, and in the moment with the other person(s), all of which are demonstrated through our non-verbal body language.

Place a check mark next to the behaviours that you typically do in conversations with others:

Open Body Language	Closed Body Language
Facing the other person	Body facing away from the other person
Looking at the other person; making some eye contact that is comfortable to you	Looking at the ground, around the room, or anywhere but at the other person
Arms unfolded, hands in lap or at sides	Arms crossed, folded over the chest
Leaning slightly towards the other person	Leaning back, away from the other person
Using some hand gestures to be congruent with your words	Staying unmoving, stoic and not having your body match what you are saying
Remaining relaxed, comfortable	Presenting as tense, uptight, or defensive

Describe the strengths you possess in communicating with others:

_____
_____
_____
_____
_____

What are your challenges in conversations with others?

_____
_____
_____
_____
_____

When you are sharing something more vulnerable and personal with others, how do you want them to act and react?

_____
_____
_____
_____
_____

How do you feel if they react this way?

_____
_____
_____

How do you feel if they react differently? How does this impact your future sharing and conversation?

_____
_____
_____
_____
_____

As the listener, it is easy to be caught up in your own thinking and to plan a response to what the other person is sharing. Truly listening, not pretending to (as many of us do), involves hearing every word that comes out of the other person's mouth, pausing to reflect on what they have said, and paraphrasing what you heard to ensure you are accurate in your interpretation.

Place a checkmark next to the strategies that you regularly use in conversation with others:

Effective Listening

Hearing every word that the other person is sharing

Not thinking about what they are saying or planning your response as they are talking

Being present in the moment

After they finish speaking, paraphrasing or reflecting back what you heard

You keep doing this until the speaker agrees, 'You have understood me'

Being empathic and understanding

What listening skills do you need to improve upon?

_____

_____

_____

_____

_____

How can you practice effective listening?

_____

_____

_____

_____

_____

Communicating effectively can take time and practice but is very rewarding and contributes to a greater depth and quality in relationships.

Verbal communication. In addition to our non-verbal communication skills of body language and listening, it is also important to pay attention to the actual words that we use and how we say them. This is our verbal communication.

What style of communicator do you tend to be?

☐ *Passive*: Those with a passive communication style are generally afraid of confrontation and do not feel they have the right to make their own wishes and desires known. They may be apologetic, deferential to others to make decisions and do not assert their needs.

☐ *Aggressive*: Aggressive communication is a method of expressing needs and desires that does not take into account the welfare of others. The aggressive communicator may appear domineering or bullying, doing anything they can to get their way in a conversation.

☐ *Passive-Aggressive*: The pattern of behaviour wherein an individual swings between the passive and aggressive communication styles depending on the moment or situation. On the surface, he/she appears passive and indifferent but in reality acts out anger in a subtle or indirect way, often through sarcasm, condescension, or patronization.

☐ *Assertive*: Communication characterized by a confident declaration or affirmation of a statement without need of proof. This affirms the person's rights or point of view without being threatening or aggressive, nor tiptoeing around the issue. The assertive individual is confident, self-aware, believes in their value as well as others', decisive, proactive, and consistent. In communication, the assertive individual embodies the healthy non-verbal communication strategies reviewed earlier and is clear and direct in expressing their needs. You may hear the assertive person say, 'I choose to ...'

When you are communicating in your typical style of communication, how do you feel?

_____
_____
_____
_____
_____

What are the biggest challenges that come up in communication for you?

_____
_____
_____
_____
_____

What changes would you like to make regarding your communication with others? List your top three goals here:

1.

2.

3.

Ideally, being an assertive communicator works best for fostering open, healthy, and functional relationships (both personally and professionally). Assertiveness requires a lot of practice with using the recovery tools and engaging honestly with others. Feedback from others is necessary to ensure that passiveness or aggressiveness are being recognized with more clarity.

Assertiveness looks like:

_____
_____
_____

_____
_____

When you are assertive, how do you feel?

_____
_____
_____
_____
_____

When we are assertive communicators, we have clear boundaries, can say 'no', and speak up for our needs in relationship with others.

What are your biggest barriers to assertiveness?

_____
_____
_____
_____
_____

Sometimes the biggest barrier to being assertive is the reaction of others, as they may not respond well when we shift our typical communication pattern. If the people in your life cannot handle this new way of being, this is confirmation that they are not healthy communicators and may not be able to be in your life in a great capacity moving forward. If they are healthy supports, then they will see that all of these changes are for the better and support you in your journey.

As you change your communication style, who has responded with anger, coldness, or detachment?

_____
_____
_____
_____
_____

How does this feel for you?

_____
_____
_____
_____
_____

What information does this give you about the relationship?

_____
_____
_____
_____
_____

As you change your communication style, who has responded with openness, support, and eagerness?

_____

_____

_____

_____

_____

How does this feel for you?

_____

_____

_____

_____

_____

What information does this give you about the relationship?

_____

_____

_____

_____

_____

As you move towards assertiveness in relationships, you can also move towards interdependence and away from enmeshment.

INTERDEPENDENCE

Interdependence is a way of defining relationships that is different than enmeshment, where all identities and needs are blended and unclear, as well as total autonomy, where identities and needs are so separate that there is no relationship. Interdependence means supporting each other to develop one's own identity, with mutual support, and relying on each other as helpers and protectors, in terms of reality checks and accountability.

What does interdependence mean to you in relationships? What does it look like?

_____

_____

_____

_____

What current relationships in your life would you describe as being interdependent?

_____

_____

_____
_____
_____

What current relationships in your life are enmeshed or autonomous?

_____
_____
_____
_____
_____

What changes would you like to see in these enmeshed or autonomous relationships?

_____
_____
_____
_____
_____

What role can you play in facilitating change in these relationships? Lay out specific steps here.

_____
_____
_____
_____
_____

Relational change can be challenging since other people are involved who may or may not be willing to grow. However, it is still possible to work on your part regardless of what changes they do or do not implement and this can have a healthy benefit to the relationship.

Key points

- There are common roles that people in families living with Addiction take on that become adaptive, a way to survive, but that may impact quality of life and relationship. It is necessary to look at your role as a family member, focus on how to move out of them to healthier ones.

- Boundaries are guidelines, rules, or limits that a person creates to identify what are reasonable, safe, and permissible ways to interact with other people around us and how we will respond when someone pushes those limits.

- The healing process for family members is just as important as for those with the disease of Addiction. There are many feelings generated for family members, which include fear, resentment, anger, guilt, and shame.

- Feelings provide us with valuable information that is necessary to listen to in order to heal emotionally and be on the path to health.

- As you move towards assertiveness in relationships, you can also move towards interdependence and away from enmeshment, codependence or Addiction involving relationships.

Action steps for Chapter 8 (follow through after chapter exercises)

In this chapter, we have explored boundaries, communication and healthy living for people who have Addiction in their family. Beyond the workbook exploration, we would encourage you to take action by continuing to learn more about the disease of Addiction and getting honest about how it has impacted you throughout your life. This can be done using community support groups, like Al-Anon, and/or in the context of professional support, like individual or group therapy. If you have Addiction in your family but do not identify having it yourself, you can still choose recovery and we hope that you will go back and complete the rest of the workbook chapters, if you have not done so already.

Chapter 9: Summary and Conclusions

"Hope is being able to see that there is light
despite all the darkness."
—*Desmond Tutu*

Our hope is that this workbook provides you greater appreciation of how Addiction as a primary, chronic brain disease impacts your life personally. We also hope that family members who are using this workbook for personal exploration are able to connect with the importance of choosing recovery for themselves, whether they have Addiction or not. With appropriate assessment and treatment of Addiction, there is hope for a better quality of life for the individual and their loved ones, more so than with other chronic diseases. Addiction is about differences in the brain functioning of people with the disease, not about their specific behaviours.

The intention of this workbook is to provide more understanding about how the brain impacts behaviour, thinking and feeling; as well as how to look at recovery along all dimensions of health (biological, psychological, social, and spiritual). This book is one tool of many in your ongoing recovery journey and in this chapter we encourage you to reflect on your journey thus far as well as continue to solidify your recovery plan.

What have been your biggest lessons and takeaways from the workbook?

_____
_____
_____
_____
_____
_____
_____

List the feelings that came up as you worked through the workbook.

_____
_____
_____
_____
_____
_____
_____

Has your personal understanding of Addiction changed as you worked through this book? How?

_____
_____
_____

_____
_____
_____
_____

There is a lot of hope in recovery for people with Addiction. Relationships grow and transform; people feel connected, serene, and peaceful; matters they once obsessed about quiet in the mind; fears lessen; cravings subside; intuition guides situations that were once baffling; trust and faith in a Higher Power develops; and life opens up a whole new realm of possibility and opportunity. These are the promises of recovery.

What are your expectations for recovery? (Note: Often expectations are "If this happens, then this will happen ...").

_____
_____
_____
_____
_____

What are your hopes for recovery? How are these different from expectations?

_____
_____
_____
_____
_____

How can you practice letting go and letting the process of recovery unfold as it needs to? What does this look like?

_____
_____
_____
_____
_____

Recovery is a day-by-day, moment-by-moment process that will unfold at its own pace and as it needs to. You need to be a responsible agent in the process by engaging in actions, behaviours, reflection, and processing regularly but it is important to remember that the disease can still have periods of greater activity that may not always be buffered by these actions.

How do you feel when your disease manifests despite your regular engagement with recovery?

_____
_____
_____
_____

It is important to not let this lead to hopelessness; it is a natural course of living with a chronic disease and it is essential to trust that recovery action is still beneficial. Regular routine and recovery structure is integral for continued health.

On a calendar, organizational app, or piece of paper, plot out your essential recovery actions for each day. It is also important to be specific about the recovery activities you will be engaging in for the week ahead.

Making your recovery the priority and having life flow around this promotes health and well-being. Over time, you will likely come to have some daily recovery routines but other activities may change as you shift. It will be important to continually re-evaluate your recovery routine to see what is working for you and what is not serving you at this time. Scheduling out recovery action for the day or week ahead is also important to prioritizing these commitments rather than letting life dictate when, where and how recovery will look.

What are your essential recovery actions at the present time?

_____

_____

_____

_____

_____

What benefit do these recovery actions provide?

_____

_____

_____

_____

_____

What recovery actions do not seem to benefit you at this time? How come they are not beneficial?

_____

_____

_____

_____

_____

It is recommended that you check out the answers to these questions with other support people in recovery, such as sponsors, recovery buddies, and your healthcare providers.

The Promises of Recovery

Recovery from Addiction has a lot to offer each individual, family, social system, society and the world. It starts with individuals choosing to do something different for themselves, knowing the brain will throw up obstacles and resistance along the way. You may not know at the beginning of your journey what the promises of recovery will be. You might read them from *The Big Book* or hear others talk about them. Even if you have yet to experience them yourself, keep trying and never give up. There is tremendous hope when it comes to recovery from Addiction and we hope everyone who uses this book gets a chance to experience that for themselves. Whether you have Addiction or not, everyone can choose recovery and benefit from it. We wish you the best in your ongoing pursuit of health, wellness and recovery.

Appendix A

RAiAR

Health Upwardly Mobile Inc. (HUM) is providing professional support to a community, peer led mutual support program called RAiAR. A RAiAR council has been established that oversees the practical logistics of starting and running RAiAR meetings in a weekly, closed small group format. Periodic open speaker meetings for new members, families and general community are part of the plan.

The small group meetings are run by peer moderators with some training in group facilitation provided by HUM. RAiAR is a complement to 12-Step and other mutual support programs, it is not a substitute. It does offer an opportunity to address all aspects of Addiction and holistic recovery in a small group discussion format, where feedback is provided in a manner where there is mutual respect and a framework of individual responsibility with accountability.

RAiAR stands for:

Remember Addiction is Addiction Responsible
...Recovery...

RAiAR has 9 steps, 9 core values, 9 slogans and 9 guiding principles, which are as follows:

- **9 steps** – willingness, action, responsible

- **9 core values** – awareness, sharing, boundaries, support, gratitude

- **9 slogans**

- **9 guiding principles** – honesty, mutual support, clarity of purpose, spiritual foundation

RAiAR Steps
Process of Recovery

1. I am willing to consider that Addiction is a primary, chronic disease that is progressive, relapsing and often causes disability and premature death.

2. I am willing to consider that Addiction manifests in biological, psychological, social and spiritual dimensions with the use of substances and/or addictive behaviours.

3. I am willing to consider that recovery is possible through support from other people and connection to a Higher Power.

4. I can and will cultivate awareness of the harm caused by my disease of addiction in my life to me and others.

5. I can and will cultivate awareness of my connection to others and my Higher Power through honest sharing.

6. I can and will actively share, from a strictly personal perspective, to surrender shame, let go of control and accept life on life's terms.

7. I am responsible for being honest and practicing humility to the best of my ability.

8. I am responsible for boundaries and balance in my life.

9. I am responsible for recovery action and staying in process, the outcomes will be determined by the grace of my Higher Power.

RAiAR Core Values

1. Life is about recognizing personal limitations and personal responsibilities.

2. Mutual support is essential for personal growth.

3. Awareness of our interconnectedness is more important than personal achievement.

4. Sharing and feedback are a process for enhancing self-awareness.

5. Sharing and feedback are always more about ourselves than other people, placesor things.

6. Responsibility for feelings and thoughts is within us, even when triggered by another person, place or thing.

7. Caring and support mean letting go of rescuing and caretaking.

8. Respect for myself and others means speaking only for myself.

9. Loving oneself and gratitude for life come before loving another person, place or thing.

RAiAR Slogans

1. Fighting feeds the disease

2. Facing feelings feeds the soul

3. Trauma is the trigger, Addiction is the trap

4. No blame, no shame

5. Recovery is a personal responsibility

6. Feedback is always a mutual process

7. Awareness not analysis

8. Remember "I" language

9. Perspectives are always personal

RAiAR Guiding Principles

1. RAiAR meetings are for people who have a desire to deal honestly with their disease of Addiction.

2. The purpose of RAiAR meetings is to support mutual growth through open sharing and caring feedback.

3. Personal recovery as experienced by individuals is the only authority in meetings, no one being more or less in authority than another.

4. Each group shall be autonomous except in matters affecting the collective purpose of RAiAR recovery.

5. The leaders shall only participate in development of guidelines and shall not govern.

6. The leaders are not teachers, experts or facilitators in the functioning of RAiAR meetings for recovery.

7. RAiAR council or committees shall have the primary purpose of service and shall be accountable to themselves and those they serve.

8. RAiAR, as a collective, shall not have any opinions or policies on outside issues.

9. RAiAR members shall individually and collectively cultivate a personal spiritual foundation for the benefit of all.

If you are looking for more information about RAiAR beyond what has already been mentioned, please contact the HUM team at info@humassociates.net

Resources for Learning More

Alcoholics Anonymous (1939). *The Big Book*. New York, NY: World Services, Inc.

Alcoholics Anonymous (1988). *Twelve steps and twelve traditions* (38th ed.). New York, NY: World Services, Inc.

Amen, D., & Smith, D. (2010). *Unchain your brain: 10 steps to breaking the addictions that steal your life*. Newport Beach, CA: Mindworks Press.

American National Institute on Drug Abuse (NIDA) (www.drugabuse.gov).

Anorexics and Bulimics Anonymous (http://aba12steps.org/).

Beattie, M. (1992). *Codependent No More*. Center City, MN: Hazelden

Bell, R.G. (1970). *Escape from Addiction*. New York, NY: McGraw-Hill Book Company.

——(1989). *A Special Calling*. Toronto, ON: Stoddart Publishing Co. Limited.

Blum, K., Oscar-Berman M., Jacobs W., McLaughlin T., Gold, M. (2014). Buprenorphine Response as a Function of Neurogenetic Polymorphic Antecedents: Can Dopamine Genes Affect Clinical Outcomes in Reward Deficiency Syndrome (RDS)? *J Addict Res Ther* 5: 185. Doi:10.4172/2155-6105.1000185.

Blum, K, Badgaiyan RD, Agan G, Fratantonio J, Simpatico T, et al. (2015). The Molecular Neurobiology of Twelve Steps Program & Fellowship: Connecting the Dots for Recovery. *J Reward Defic Syndr* 1(1): 46–64.

Brown, B. (2007). *I thought it was just me (but it isn't): Making the journey from 'what will people think?' to 'I am enough.'* New York, NY: Penguin Group.

Brown, B. (2009). *Connections: A 12-session psychoeducational shame-resilience curriculum*. Center City, MN: Hazelden.

Brown, B. (2010). *The gifts of imperfection*. Center City, MN: Hazelden.

Codependents Anonymous (www.coda.org)

Doran, G. T. (1981). There's a S.M.A.R.T. way to write management's goals and objectives. *Management Review*, 70(11), 35–36.

DuPont, R. L. (2000). *The selfish brain: Learning from Addiction*. Center City, MN: Hazelden.

Edenberg, H. J. (2011, September 9). *Genetics of alcoholism*. Presented at the World Congress of Psychiatric Genetics symposium on The Genetics and Epigenetics of Substance Abuse. Presentation retrieved February 7, 2015 from www.drugabuse.gov/news-events/meetings-events/2011/09/genetics-epigenetics-substance-abuse

Fletcher, B.W., Chandler, R.K. (2006). *Principles of Drug Abuse Treatment for Criminal Justice Populations*. Washington, DC: National Institute on Drug Abuse. NIH publication 06–5316. Retrieved February 6, 2015 from www.drugabuse.gov/sites/default/files/txcriminaljustice_0.pdf

The Foundation for Addiction and Mental Health (www.famh.ca)

Hajela, R., Newton, S., & Abbott, P. (2015). *Addiction is Addiction: Understanding the disease in oneself and others for a better quality of life* (1st ed.) Victoria, BC: FriesenPress.

HBO Addiction Project (2007). www.drugabuse.gov/news-events/public/hbo-addiction-project. Retrieved July 14, 2014 from www.hbo.com

Karpman, S. (1968). Fairy tales and script drama analysis. *Transactional Analysis Bulletin, 7* (26), 39–43.

Jellinek, E. M. (1960). *The Disease Concept of Alcoholism.* New Haven, CT: Hillhouse.

Kendler, K. (2011, September 9). *The genetic epidemiology of substance abuse.* Presented at the World Congress of Psychiatric Genetics symposium on The Genetics and Epigenetics of Substance Abuse. Presentation retrieved February 7, 2015 from www.drugabuse.gov/news-events/meetings-events/2011/09/genetics-epigenetics-substance-abuse

Linehan, M. M. (2014). *Skills training manual for treating borderline personality disorder* (2nd ed.). New York, NY: Guilford Press.

Luft, J., & Ingham, H. (1955). *The Johari window, a graphic model of interpersonal awareness.* Presented at the Proceedings of the Western Training Laboratory in Group Development. Retrieved May 29, 2014 from http://www.businessballs.com/johariwindowmodel.htm

Mee-Lee, D. (Ed.) (2013). *The ASAM criteria: Treatment criteria for addictive, substance-related, and co-occurring conditions* (3rd ed.). Carson City, NV: The Change Companies.

Miller, W. R., & Rollnick, S. (2012). *Motivational interviewing: Helping people change* (3rd ed.). New York, NY: Guilford Press.

Miller, W. R., & Rose, G. S. (2009). Toward a theory of motivational interviewing. *American Psychologist, 64*(6), 527–537.

Mooney, A. J., Dold, C. & Eisenberg H. (2014) *The Recovery Book: Answers to All Your Questions About Addiction and Alcoholism and Finding Health and Happiness in Sobriety* (2nd ed.). New York, NY: Workman Publishing.

The National Center on Addiction and Substance Abuse (CASA). (2012). *CASA Columbia analysis of the National Survey on Drug Use and Health (NSDUH).* Rockville, MD: U.S. Department of Health and Human Services, Substance Abuse and Mental Health Services Administration.

National Institute on Drug Abuse (2014). *Drugs, brains and behaviour: The science of Addiction.* Retrieved February 7, 2015 from http://www.drugabuse.gov/sites/default/files/soa_2014.pdf

Nestler, E. (2011, September 9). *Epigenetics of addiction.* Presented at the World Congress of Psychiatric Genetics symposium on The Genetics and Epigenetics of Substance Abuse. Abstract retrieved February 7, 2015 from http://www.drugabuse.gov/news-events/meetings-events/2011/09/genetics-epigenetics-substance-abuse

Nicols, M. P. (2012). *Family therapy: Concepts and methods* (10th ed.). Upper Saddle River, NJ: Pearson Press.

Prochaska, J. O., & DiClemente, C. C. (2005). The transtheoretical approach. In J. C. Norcross, M. R. Goldfried (Eds.). *Handbook of psychotherapy integration* (2nd ed.) (pp. 147–171). New York, NY: Oxford University Press.

Schaef, A. W. (1987) *When Society Becomes An Addict.* New York, NY: Harper & Row Publisher.

Sex Addicts Anonymous (www.saa-recovery.org).

Sex and Love Addicts Anonymous (www.slaafws.org)

Sexaholics Anonymous (www.sa.org).

Twerski, A. J. (1982). *It happens to doctors, too.* Center City, MN: Hazelden.

——(1997). *Addictive thinking: Understanding self-deception* (2nd ed.). Center City, MN: Hazelden.

Vaillant, G. (2005). Alcoholics Anonymous: Cult or cure? *Australian and New Zealand Journal of Psychiatry, 39,* 431–436.

Wegsheider-Cruse, S. (1986). *Choicemaking: For Spirituality Seekers, Co-dependents and Adult Children.* Pompano Beach, FL: ealth Communications Incorporated.

Yalom, I. (2002). *The gift of therapy: An open letter to a new generation of therapists and their patients.* New York, NY: Harper Collins.

About the Authors

Ms. Sue Newton is a principal of Health Upwardly Mobile Inc. and the vice president and operations director since its founding in 2009. She has been a registered nurse since 1988 and completed both her Bachelor of Arts degree in Psychology and Bachelor of Science in Nursing from Lakehead University in 1988 and received her Master's degree in Nursing from the University of Calgary in 1996. Sue initially worked for Alberta Health Services for nineteen years in both acute care and public health in a number of clinical and management roles. In 2008, she left Alberta Health Services to work as the nurse manager for an integrated health and wellness company in Calgary focusing on Occupational Health and an employee and family assistance program (EFAP). Sue started doing transcendental meditation in 2010 and continues to meditate regularly. She also became a certified yoga instructor in 2015, her focus is on Critical Alignment Yoga Therapy.

Ms. Paige Abbott is the clinical services director at Health Upwardly Mobile Inc. She has been a registered psychologist since 2009 and she completed her Master of Science degree in Counselling Psychology at the University of Calgary in 2007. After graduation, Paige worked at an employee and family assistance program (EFAP) from 2008–2012. During her time at the EFAP agency, she worked as a staff psychologist and took on the additional role as manager of a number of different programs, including crisis management services, wellness and workshops, and professional services in Southern Alberta. Paige has been a member of the HUM team since 2011. Paige engages in a number of daily and regular recovery actions. Her current go-tos are meditation, journalling, social connection, yoga and connection to the universe.

Dr. Raju Hajela is a principal of Health Upwardly Mobile Inc. (HUM) and the president and medical director. HUM was founded in 2009 as a health and wellness company in Calgary, Alberta, Canada, which specializes in Addiction, mental health, chronic pain and occupational health. Raju received his MD from Dalhousie University in 1982 and his Master of Public Health from the Harvard School of Public Health in 1988. Raju served in the Canadian Forces from 1979 to 1995. He has specialized training and extensive experience in Addiction, mental health, chronic pain, and occupational health. He has held leadership positions in provincial, national, and international medical organizations. Raju has been a Transcendental Meditation practitioner since 1986. He has received training in Maharishi Ayurveda and advanced meditation techniques.

CPSIA information can be obtained
at www.ICGtesting.com
Printed in the USA
LVHW05s2230130618
580522LV00016B/107/P